10-8-2)
04

The "I hate to exercise" BOOK

for people with diabetes

by Charlotte Hayes, MMSc, MS, RD, CDE

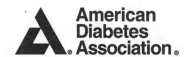
American
Diabetes
Association.

Director, Book Publishing, John Fedor; *Associate Director, Consumer Book Acquisitions,* Sherrye Landrum; *Editor,* Abe Ogden; *Production Manager,* Peggy M. Rote; *Composition,* Circle Graphics, Inc.; *Cover Design,* KSA Plus Communications; *Printer,* Port City Press, Inc.

Printed in the United States of America
1 3 5 7 9 10 8 6 4 2

The suggestions and information contained in this publication are generally consistent with the *Clinical Practice Recommendations* and other policies of the American Diabetes Association, but they do not represent the policy or position of the Association or any of its boards or committees. Reasonable steps have been taken to ensure the accuracy of the information presented. However, the American Diabetes Association cannot ensure the safety or efficacy of any product or service described in this publication. Individuals are advised to consult a physician or other appropriate health care professional before undertaking any diet or exercise program or taking any medication referred to in this publication. Professionals must use and apply their own professional judgment, experience, and training and should not rely solely on the information contained in this publication before prescribing any diet, exercise, or medication. The American Diabetes Association—its officers, directors, employees, volunteers, and members—assumes no responsibility or liability for personal or other injury, loss, or damage that may result from the suggestions or information in this publication.

♾ The paper in this publication meets the requirements of the ANSI Standard Z39.48-1992 (permanence of paper).

ADA titles may be purchased for business or promotional use or for special sales. For information, please write to Lee Romano Sequeira, Special Sales & Promotions, at the address below.

American Diabetes Association
1701 North Beauregard Street
Alexandria, Virginia 22311

Library of Congress Cataloging-in-Publication Data

Hayes, Charlotte, 1958–
   The "I hate to exercise" book for people with diabetes / Charlotte Hayes.
     p. cm.
   Includes index.
   ISBN 1-58040-044-2 (pbk. : alk. paper)
    1. Diabetes—Exercise therapy. I. Title

RC661.E94 H34 2001
616.4'62062—dc21

                                              2001022095

Contents

1

Why Should You Care About Exercise?

Good for you. Opening the book counts. It burned a few calories. In fact, doing just about any activity burns calories. For instance, people who fidget burn more calories than people who just sit. So, wiggle your foot, tap your fingers, rock in a rocking chair. When you're moving, you're burning calories—which is a goal of nearly every person in our society.

But fidgeting isn't really exercise. It won't bring you all the benefits that you want from exercise. So, what do you do? Perhaps you hate exercise because you don't know how to do it. Perhaps the word exercise brings up a painful or embarrassing memory of junior high gym class. Perhaps you're too overweight and out of shape even to imagine yourself getting up and doing anything. Well, the good news is; you've got a friend. This book will show you that you really are already doing things that count as exercise—things you enjoy much more than gym class or fidgeting. And this book can tell you how to add activity to your day—and maybe no one else will even know that you are exercising!

So what you're really asking is: how can I become a person who exercises—and enjoys it? Read on.

Why Exercise?

Exercise is the magic bullet—the perfect pill—the solution to most health problems.

People spend hours and many dollars shopping for the perfect outfits to make themselves look good, when if they spent as little as thirty minutes a day, they could make their bodies look good in anything they put on. Exercise is all it's cracked up to be. Exercise:

- lifts your mood
- lightens your weight
- builds muscles which burn calories even at REST
- reduces stress, anxiety, and depression
- improves your sex life
- gives you MORE energy
- makes you feel great
- makes you look great
- makes you proud of yourself

There is a strong link between "sitting" your way through life and developing many of the chronic diseases we struggle with today:

- heart disease
- high blood pressure
- high blood fat levels
- obesity and overweight
- type 2 diabetes

Chances are that if you already have type 2 diabetes, you also have one or more of these other conditions, too—or you are at a higher risk of developing them. Is that why you're reading this book? What can you do to prevent or control these conditions? Well, no pill can do it, but exercise can. Like a magic wand, you can transform your body, your health, and you. Exercise works on all these health problems equally well—and unlike most pills, it works without side effects.

Wait! There's more. Exercise improves your self-image. Exercise postpones aging. In fact, with exercise you can move gracefully through all your years with the flexibility and strength to do the things you need to do—and want to do—for yourself. With exercise, you have a better quality of life all the way through.

So, why are so many people inactive?

We don't have to move much any more. Many of the chores and activities that filled our daily lives with exercise have been erased by modern technology. Elevators, dishwashers, washing machines, riding lawn mowers, remote controls—inventions like these have made our lives easier. Unfortunately, they've made our lives so easy that we must now take steps to increase our activity if we want to stay healthy. Our bodies are like our machines—they must be used to stay in good working condition.

Okay, now comes the groaning part—and all those excuses for why you don't exercise. Simply put, most people say they don't exercise because they have no time, no place, or no one to go with them. Or they're afraid to start because they've never done it before—or it's those memories of high school gym class. What's your excuse?

Is there another way?

Yes. You don't have to change jobs or give up your free time to fit exercise into your schedule. You don't have to go to the gym or jog every day. In fact, you never have to do those things. The latest research has found that physical activity does not need to be vigorous or structured to be good for you. Everyday chores, work-related tasks, and leisure-time activities count, too. In 1996 the Surgeon General of the United States offered this guideline on activity to improve your health.

"Every adult in the U.S. should accumulate 30 minutes or more of moderate-intensity physical activity on most, preferably all, days of the week."

What this means is that you don't have to go out and exercise for a long stretch of time. You can do small amounts of activities during the day that add up to 30 minutes. Five minutes of walking three times a day plus 15 minutes of running the vacuum cleaner adds up to your 30 minutes. Are those physical activities? That's the best part. Doing enjoyable activities that fit into your daily life—such as brisk walking, yard work, gardening, and household chores—is as good for you as structured and vigorous exercise. In fact, in one study, the group of women who gardened several days each week had greater bone mass than walkers and joggers, so don't discount any physical activity as not being vigorous enough because it doesn't work up a sweat. Sweating is not required.

If you haven't been very active up to this point, don't worry. It's never too late. In fact, people in their 90s who start lifting 1-pound weights put on muscle just like 20-somethings do. There are a lot of health myths about what aging does to physical ability. Don't believe any of them. Just keep it simple. Begin with a few minutes of physical activity each day—really, no more than 5 minutes to start. Build up gradually to doing a total of 30 minutes. Add a minute or two each week. Don't get in a hurry or you may get too sore to enjoy yourself, or you might injure yourself. Slow and steady wins the race, remember? If you have been doing some activity—such as walking—but haven't been doing it every day, try to add a few minutes each time or start doing it every day. The amount of activity you do is more important than what you do. And doing something is always better than sitting there and thinking about it.

What if you have diabetes?

Everyone can succeed at becoming fit and healthy. Yes, even you. Having diabetes makes it even more important for you to be physically active. Exercise improves your body's ability to use insulin, and this improves your diabetes control in many ways. Physical activity also helps relieve stress, lift depression, and brighten your mood. When you have a chronic disease, this can make a huge difference. Exercise builds muscle, and muscle burns calories even at rest. There is nothing better than exercise because it just keeps on improving your health!

Exercise your way to blood glucose control

If you have type 2 diabetes, regular activity improves your blood glucose control. Exercise lowers blood glucose levels because it takes glucose out of the blood to use for energy during and after exercise. It also helps lower blood glucose levels in other ways:

- Muscle cells become more sensitive to insulin, so they do a better job of storing and using glucose for energy.

- Liver cells become more sensitive to insulin, preventing the liver from producing too much glucose.
- Exercise increases the amount of muscle you have. Muscle uses glucose as an energy source even while you're at rest. More muscle means lower glucose!
- Exercise helps you lose weight—and keep it off. No more yo-yo weight loss. If you are overweight, a loss of even 10 to 20 pounds can really improve blood glucose readings.

Exercise your way to a healthy heart

If you are inactive, you are at greater risk for developing heart disease. If you also have diabetes, your chances of developing heart disease are even more alarming. Regular physical activity works in several ways to keep your heart healthy.

- It strengthens your heart muscle. A strong heart does a better job of pumping blood throughout your body. This is especially important at times of stress when the demands on your heart are high.
- It lowers your resting heart rate. This reduces work for your heart.
- It lowers blood pressure. This also reduces work for your heart.
- It lowers total cholesterol levels, increases HDL (good) cholesterol, and lowers triglyceride levels in the blood. This reduces the risk that important arteries in your heart will become blocked.
- It may act as a natural blood thinner, much like aspirin, and may help reduce the risk of heart attack and stroke.

Exercise your way to weight control

Weight loss is often an important goal for people with diabetes, especially those with type 2. Losing even a small amount of weight can improve your blood glucose levels. For some people with diabetes, dropping some pounds may mean that they can stop taking insulin and other diabetes medications and control the disease with diet and exercise alone. Too often, however, people try to lose weight just by cutting back on what they eat. They don't increase their activity at the same time. But the pounds come off faster and stay off if you add exercise to meal planning. In fact, exercising when you're trying to lose weight:

- Helps promote fat loss and prevent muscle loss. You naturally lose muscle as you age, so exercise helps you hold on to it.
- Boosts your metabolic rate. This means your body burns calories as heat instead of storing them as fat.
- Helps you burn extra calories. For example, if you walk 3 miles in an hour, you may burn about 300 calories—or the full meal you enjoyed for breakfast. If you sit in a chair for an hour, you will burn only about 60 calories—so you only need half a piece of toast for breakfast.
- Helps reduce excess weight around your middle. Although it's not possible to "spot reduce," when you lose weight overall, you often lose pounds around your middle. Losing weight in this area is especially important for reducing blood pressure, improving blood fat levels, and improving blood glucose levels.
- Helps reduce your appetite.
- Helps reduce stress and anxiety that can lead to overeating. If you overeat as a way to cope with stress, you'll find that exercise is a better coping mechanism in many ways.

So, the good news is that when you add exercise to your life you can improve your blood glucose control and your general health AND lose weight. And you don't even have to go to a fitness center or do vigorous exercise to do it! You can get the same benefits just by fitting moderate activity into your daily routine.

What do you do first?

So, you want all the benefits being active can give you. Now what? First, talk with your doctor and diabetes educators about your desire to increase your level of activity. They should support you in this effort and help you come up with safe and enjoyable ways of increasing your activity level. Your doctor will probably want you to have a thorough check-up before you begin exercising, especially if you have complications of diabetes. The doctor may want to check you over if you:

- are over 35 years old
- have had type 2 diabetes for more than 10 years
- have had type 1 diabetes for more than 15 years
- have high blood pressure
- have high blood fat levels
- have heart disease
- have poor circulation in your feet or legs
- have retinopathy (diabetic eye disease)
- have neuropathy (diabetic nerve damage—symptoms include numbness, tingling, or loss of feeling in the feet; blood pressure drop when moving from sitting to standing; lack of sweating; and not being able to sense low blood sugar)
- have nephropathy (diabetic kidney disease)
- have a family history of premature coronary artery disease (CAD)

If you have complications of diabetes, some activities may be safer for you to do than others, and the way you do the activities may be modified so you can perform them safely. This is especially true if you consider doing a higher-intensity activity. Table 1-1 lists activities to be cautious about doing if you have diabetes-related complications; it also gives some safe, alternative activities. Most moderate lifestyle activities—the type that the Surgeon General encourages you to fit into your daily routine—are safe to do when you have complications of diabetes. So, don't consider your diabetes a barrier to becoming more active.

Looking at Your Lifestyle

Once your doctor gives you the okay to become more active, take time to look at your lifestyle. Try to find ways around any exercise obstacles that trip you up and get rid of the bad habits that have been keeping you from a healthy

Table 1-1 Exercising Safely with Diabetes Complications

DIABETES COMPLICATION	CAUTION!	BENEFICIAL ACTIVITIES
Heart disease	Very strenuous activity	Moderate activity such as walking, daily chores, gardening, fishing
	Heavy lifting or straining, isometric exercises	Moderate dynamic lifting, stretching
	Exercise in extreme heat or cold	Activity in a moderate climate
High blood pressure	Very strenuous activity Heavy lifting or straining and isometric exercise	Most moderate activity such as walking, moderate lifting, weight lifting with light weights and high repetitions, stretching
Nephropathy (also refer to blood pressure guidelines)	Strenuous activity	Light to moderate daily activities such as walking, light household chores, gardening, water exercise
Neuropathy	Weight bearing activities especially if high impact, strenuous, or prolonged such as: walking a distance, treadmill exercise, step exercise, jumping/hopping, exercise in heat or cold	Moderate activities that are low impact (e.g. cycling, swimming, chair exercises, stretching), light to moderate daily activities, exercise in a moderate climate
Retinopathy	Strenuous exercise, activities that require heavy lifting and straining, breath holding while lifting or pushing, isometric exercise, high impact activities that cause jarring, head-low activities	Moderate activities that are low impact (e.g. walking, cycling, water exercise), moderate daily chores that do not involve heavy lifting, straining, or the head to be lower than the waist
Peripheral vascular disease	High impact activities	Moderate walking (may do intermittent exercise with periods of walking followed by periods of rest), non-weight bearing exercise: swimming, cycling, chair exercises
Osteoporosis or arthritis	High impact activities	Moderate daily activities, walking, water exercise, resistance exercise (e.g. light lifting activities), stretching

lifestyle. Most important, try to enlist the help of supportive people in your life.

How do you manage your time?

One of the great things about physical activity is that it can fit naturally into your day. Look at your daily routine to pinpoint times when you can realistically take a few minutes to do some activity. Ten minutes here or there can make a big difference. For example, you can:

- get up 10 minutes earlier than usual and do some stretches
- park at the far end of the parking lot and walk for 10 minutes
- use the stairs instead of the elevator 4 or 5 times a day
- take a 10-minute stroll after lunch to burn calories
- spend 10 minutes stretching when you get home from work

A little planning ahead allows you to slip activity into your day with ease. Of course, you need to be honest. If you hate getting up early, don't schedule any exercise time then. You'll hate the exercise, too, and you won't do it. Holidays, vacations, or demanding times with work or family can squeeze your time and make extra planning necessary. When you have to cut back, remind yourself that doing something, even if it's less than usual, is always better than doing nothing. Keep moving as a gift to yourself that truly does keep on giving.

Smoking

You don't need a doctor to tell you that cigarette smoking does not fit in a vigorous and healthy lifestyle. Smoking not only harms your health all by itself, it can make becoming physically active unpleasant, even painful. For example, if you smoke, you may have great difficulty climbing a flight of stairs and find yourself panting heavily before you reach the top. The immediate discomfort you feel could keep you from taking the stairs the next time and send you right back to the elevator. If you can cut back on smoking—or better yet, kick your habit completely—you'll be surprised at how good you feel and how much easier and more enjoyable physical activity becomes.

Eating

Eating well is essential to good health and definitely influences how we feel and how well we function. Athletes and avid exercisers often talk about how important diet and nutrition are for achieving peak performance. Healthy food is premium fuel for your body. Though most of us are not athletes, healthy eating is still necessary for good health, well being, and our best daily performance. Healthy eating is also a cornerstone of good diabetes management. If your eating habits have been iffy, you may have poor diabetes control and sagging energy. Donuts won't get you as far as oatmeal. Healthy eating and physical activity are a powerful pair. Together, they can lead to improvements in blood glucose readings, blood fat levels, blood pressure, and weight. As your diabetes control and overall health improve, you'll begin to feel more energized and ready to be more physically active.

Gaining support from others

You need support. It's great to have someone to walk with. And it's great to have someone tell you how great you are for exercising. Involving supportive people in your exercise plan can spread the benefits around. Your family members, friends, neighbors, and co-workers can all reap the health benefits of being active and joining you. Exercising with others is motivating and can be a lot of fun. In fact, the fun and social aspects of doing activity with others can be what helps you stick with your plan at times when you don't feel like exercising. Phone calls and friendly reminders from others, who count on you to be there too, can provide the extra nudge that is necessary for success. And if you know someone who is committed to living a physically active lifestyle and has established a consistent activity routine, ask them for guidance and support as you are becoming more active. A good role model can understand the challenges you face, provide feedback about the progress you have made, and offer helpful suggestions about how to succeed with your activity goals.

Even if the significant people in your life do not participate in the activity themselves, you need their support. Sometimes you'll need to ask others to rearrange their schedules so that you can fit physical activity into yours. If you plan to exercise early in the morning, for example, you might ask your spouse to prepare breakfast. You may ask co-workers whether they can be flexible about their lunch schedules so that you can walk during your lunch break. Enlisting support before you set activity goals is a good idea so that everyone can agree ahead of time on a plan that allows you to fit activity into your routine.

2

What's Your Goal?

Just do it! You've probably heard that before, but it's the first step toward success with becoming physically active. However, don't do it all at once. For example, if you plan to hike 3 miles up a mountain for your first attempt at exercise, you'll probably come home discouraged. A more realistic way to start would be to walk to the end of your block and home again. By being kinder and gentler with realistic expectations of what you can accomplish, your first activity session will be much more enjoyable and successful. You'll feel energized by the activity rather than completely worn out, and you'll feel good when you are done rather than relieved that the chore is over. Best of all, you'll experience a sense of satisfaction because you have done what you set out to do.

That feeling of accomplishment is very important when you are starting to increase activity. And when you have reasonable expectations of what you can do and set goals that you can achieve, success is sure to follow. Experiencing success is not only satisfying, it is very encouraging: It will help you establish a commitment to just do it—and to keep on doing it.

Setting Activity Goals

Setting goals can help you make gradual, steady progress toward increasing your activity level. With many things we do in daily life, we create a "plan of attack." Take baking a loaf of bread, for example. You want to bake a loaf of French

13

bread for Sunday dinner—that's your overall goal. Your plan of attack would include buying the ingredients, deciding what time of day to start making the bread in order to have it ready by dinnertime, and then following a recipe step-by-step so that you end up with a delicious loaf. It's much the same when you set a goal for increasing physical activity: It's not enough to say, "I will begin walking regularly." A goal that includes a plan of attack would be more specific, such as, "I will walk for 20 minutes three times a week on my lunch hour with my friend Rose."

Below are a few guidelines for goal setting and creating a plan of attack. When you set goals:

Be specific
- decide what you want to accomplish
- where you will do the activity
- when you will do the activity
- how you will do the activity
- who will support you in your goal

Be realistic
- keep the amount of activity you plan to do at a comfortable level
- be confident that you can accomplish what you set out to do

Think short term
- set daily or weekly goals
- make sure your short-term goals guide you toward your long-term goal of active living

Be flexible
- as circumstances change, be willing to modify or reset goals
- be willing to find new alternatives to challenging situations
- avoid "all or none" thinking

Reward yourself for accomplishing goals
- rewards should be meaningful
- rewards should reinforce your goal

To illustrate how you can set goals properly, let's create a fictional character—Gloria—and see how she used goal setting to successfully start a daily activity routine. Gloria has type 2 diabetes. Like a lot of people, she did very little physical activity of any kind. At work she mostly sat at a computer. In the evening, she did some light household chores and watched TV. Gloria realized that she would be healthier and feel better if she lost a few pounds and got her blood sugar under good control. She read a pamphlet in her doctor's office about the health benefits of moderate daily activity and decided she would like to build up to doing 30 minutes of activity every day. But because she was out of shape, Gloria had trouble imagining how she would ever be able to actually do this.

To overcome the biggest hurdle of all—getting started—Gloria decided to make a plan. This is how she got started:

Since she wasn't used to vigorous exercise, Gloria knew that doing 30 minutes of activity every day was probably too much for her to start out with. Instead, she thought about what she could realistically do tomorrow. She felt quite sure that she could comfortably do two activity sessions, each lasting for 3 to 5 minutes. She knew that the activity should feel good and be energizing; it should not be so tiring and painful that the thought of exercise made her cringe.

Gloria decided to take a "one day at a time" and "one week at a time" approach. She knew that by thinking short-term she could build up step-by-step to doing 30 minutes of daily activity. She also knew that by taking this approach she could achieve small victories along the way and this would encourage her to keep going.

Next, Gloria developed a specific plan for the coming week:

"I will do 3 to 5 minutes of activity twice a day at least four days next week. I will walk for 3 to 5 minutes at the beginning of my lunch break and will do 3 to 5 minutes of chair exercises during my TV program at night. I will tell my co-workers that I am going to walk at lunchtime and will ask them to join me. I will tell my husband that I plan to do an activity session at home during the evenings. I will ask him to join me and work with me to become more physically active."

By allowing herself to achieve her exercise goal just four out of seven days, Gloria knew she was creating a flexible plan and was avoiding "all or nothing" thinking. If she didn't manage to be active every day, there was room for this, and she wouldn't feel like she was breaking away from her plan.

Gloria enjoyed getting a manicure on Saturdays but had always considered this to be a bit of a luxury. As a reward for accomplishing her weekly activity goal, Gloria decided to treat herself to a manicure only if she stuck to her activity plan.

Gloria did establish an activity habit and worked up to doing 30 minutes of activity on most days. It took her several months to get to that level, but by setting realistic, short-term goals she made gradual progress, enjoyed the activity that she did, and successfully accomplished what she had hoped to do. In addition, Gloria's blood glucose control and blood fat levels improved, and she lost some weight, too. Best of all, she felt better and more energetic—and enjoyed the satisfaction of her success!

Strategies for Success

Setting goals and making a plan to achieve them are first steps toward committing yourself to exercise. But staying committed is another thing altogether. If you tried to maintain an exercise regimen before, you know how difficult it is to stick to your plan. What follows are some strategies for keeping yourself on track in achieving your fitness goals.

Make a contract with yourself

A good way to stay on track is to make your commitment more concrete. A physical activity contract is a written and signed agreement that states your activity goals and how you plan to accomplish them. The purpose of the contract is to help you stay committed to increasing physical activity and to remain focused while you work to reach your goals. It is an agreement that you make with yourself, so once you write the contract, you sign it. You might ask a friend or other supportive person to sign it as well. The idea here is that when you involve another person in your contract, you not only make a public statement about your activity goals, you ask the other person to help you uphold your agreement with yourself. (But remind the other person that nagging is not part of the job!) This adds weight to your contract, increases your sense of commitment, and, ahead of time, enlists the help of individuals you can turn to if you have difficulty achieving your goals. A well-written contract:

- states your specific activity goals
- formalizes your plan of action for achieving your goals
- sets a time frame
- identifies how you will reward yourself
- is signed and dated

Figure 2-1 shows a sample physical activity contract. Now, let's go back to our example, Gloria, and see how she used this contract.

1. Gloria decided on a reasonable time-frame for accomplishing her goal(s): This is a 1-week contract. I will begin working toward the goals stated in this contract on June 16, and I will evaluate my progress toward achieving these goals on June 23.
2. Gloria then stated her specific physical activity goal for the next week: Goal # 1: I will do 3 to 5 minutes of physical activity twice a day at least 4 days next week.
3. She then defined how she was going to accomplish this goal: My Plan of Action—Goal #1:
   A. I will walk for between 3 and 5 minutes at the beginning of my lunch break at least 2 out of 5 days next week or
   B. I will do chair exercises for 3 to 5 minutes during my evening TV program at least 2 out of 7 nights next week.
4. Gloria wrote down how she would reward herself when she achieved her goal: I will have a manicure on Saturday afternoon as a reward for achieving my activity goal.

Figure 2-1 Sample Lifestyle Activity Contract

Lifestyle Activity Contract

Duration/Time-frame of agreement:

This is a _____ week contract. I will begin working toward the goals stated in this contract on _____ and I will evaluate my progress toward achieving these goals on _____.

My Goal(s):

1. _____

2. _____

3. _____

My Plan of Action:

Goal 1: _____

Goal 2: _____

Goal 3: _____

My Reward for Achieving My Goal(s):

_____

Signed:

_____   _____
YOUR SIGNATURE   DATE

_____   _____
SUPPORTIVE OTHER SIGNATURE   DATE

5. Gloria gained the support of her husband and a friend at work. She signed and dated the contract and asked each of them to sign it to show their support.

With her signed physical activity contract in hand, Gloria was a step closer toward realizing her fitness goals.

Keeping self-talk positive

Self-talk is the inner conversation that we all have with ourselves. This conversation is not only a reflection of our thoughts and emotions; it also has a strong influence on how successful we are at making lifestyle changes. Self-talk that is positive and upbeat leads to success; self-talk that is negative and distorted can get in your way. That's why it's so important to be aware of the conversations you have with yourself about physical activity. If you tell yourself, "I've never been able to stick with exercise. I guess I'm just too lazy to be in good shape," you are being too hard on yourself and giving yourself an excuse for failure.

Sometimes it is helpful to consider where such negative thoughts come from. Maybe you were the kind of person who never had much success with sports, the kind of person that took four years of home economics to stay out of gym class. Perhaps this formed your thinking about your ability to be physically active as an adult. The good news is that you can turn negative self-talk into realistic positive reinforcement. A healthy statement that is self-supporting might be, "I know that I'm no marathon runner and that's alright. Gardening and walking are activities I enjoy, and I can improve my health by doing them." Table 2-1 lists some discouraging thoughts that might seem familiar and offers examples of how to turn those negative conversations into positive pep talks. If you catch yourself having a negative internal conversation about exercise, remember that you have the ability to turn things around. Talk back to yourself with a positive response.

Is the effort worth the result?

Very seldom are things in life absolutely free. Even if you are fortunate enough to win the lottery, first you had to buy a ticket. When some people weigh the low cost of the ticket against the possibility of winning big, they decide the investment is worth the risk. Others figure that the chances of winning are so slim that the cost of a ticket is just money down the drain.

Every day we make many similar cost/benefit decisions, especially when we think about making lifestyle changes. If we see the cost as being reasonable and the benefit—or what we'll get in return—as being worth it, we tend to buy into the idea of making changes. But if the cost seems too high and the benefits are uncertain, we usually aren't as likely to

Table 2-1 Distorted Thoughts and Positive Alternatives

TYPE OF DISTORTED THOUGHT	EXAMPLE	POSITIVE ALTERNATIVE
All or nothing thinking	I didn't walk every day last week. I'm an exercise failure.	I walked 4 out of 7 days last week; every time I do some activity I make progress toward my goal.
Disqualifying the positive	The only reason I parked far away from the entrance to the store was because I couldn't find a close parking spot.	I'm glad I decided to park at the end of the parking lot because I was able to do some extra walking on the way into the store.
Overgeneralization	I can't run, so I can't get enough exercise to do me any good.	I like to walk; it is a good, healthy activity for me to do.
Negative interpretation	My doctor wants me to have a foot evaluation before I start doing more activity. That must mean exercise is bad for my feet.	Because I have diabetes, I always have to take very good care of my feet. I'm glad that my doctor is making sure that the activity I do is right for me.
Personalization	The weatherman has something against me. I was planning to walk, but it has been raining cats and dogs all day long. I just can't win.	You can never really predict the weather, so I'm glad I have a plan for doing exercise indoors on rainy days like today.

make the effort. For this reason, doing a cost/benefit analysis—which really amounts to listing the pros and cons of the situation to see if the effort is worth the result—before you make a lifestyle change can be a helpful exercise.

A sample cost/benefit analysis appears in Table 2-2. To start your own analysis, first list things that you consider to be the costs—or cons—about doing more activity. Some examples might include:

- the extra time it will take
- the need to change your routine
- the sore muscles or other discomfort you might experience
- the notion that you just don't like doing activity

Then list all the benefits—or pros—of making the change, the things that you will gain from being more active. Such benefits might include:

- feeling better
- looking better
- improved health and diabetes control
- increased energy level
- better mood
- the ability to do more of the things you want to do

Now, weigh the pros and cons, and think of ways to reduce the costs and increase the benefits. For example, you can help avoid muscle soreness by setting realistic activity goals and gradually working up to them. And you can make time for exercise by setting your alarm clock a little earlier each day. Ultimately, your aim is to have a balance sheet that is long on benefits and short on costs—and that makes you a winner!

Giving yourself cues

Cues are signals that trigger us to take action. An actor, for example, depends on cues to tell him the correct time to come onstage. A traffic light that turns red is a cue that tells us to stop the car. Advertisers target TV viewers with numerous cues in commercials. If you find your mouth watering in response to an ad for a piping-hot pizza, you are responding to a powerful food cue. This cue may send you straight to the refrigerator or to the phone to call for carry-out.

Cues can be positive and helpful or they can be negative and obstructive (if you are trying to lose weight, for example, the pizza commercial could be bad news for your diet). And they can definitely influence your success with doing activity. For example, if you plan to walk after work, putting your walking shoes just inside the front door can serve as a positive cue: When you see them, that's your reminder to walk. On the other hand, if the first thing you see when you get home is a comfortable chair and a TV remote, this can be a negative cue. You may find yourself plopping down in front of the tube instead of going for a pleasant walk.

Table 2-2 Sample Physical Activity Cost/Benefit Balance Sheet

COST	HOW SIGNIF-ICANT	STRATEGIES TO DECREASE	BENEFIT	HOW SIGNIF-ICANT	STRATEGIES TO INCREASE
Time	V	Do small amounts of activity at convenient times	Better health	V	Do regular activity
			Feel better	V	Be moderate and consistent
Discomfort	M	Keep activity light/moderate and comfortable	More energy	V	Gradually increase activity
Boredom	M	Do a variety of activities to gain fitness	Greater ability to do things I enjoy	V	Gradually "build up" to get stronger
Inconvenience	M	Fit activity into work and home routine	Look better	M	Increase activity enough to lose weight and gain muscle
Embarrassment	M	Do only what I know I can successfully do	Enjoyment	V	Do activity with friends; do outside activities on nice days
Unenjoyable	M	Be open minded and try different activities to find some I like	Time with friends	M	Arrange to do activity with friends
Expense	NV	Do activities at home that don't require special equipment	Manage stress	V	Plan activity "stress breaks" of stretching or walking
Place to exercise	NV	Find ways to do activity at work or at home	Like the challenge	M	Set goals that are challenging but within reach

Significance Key: V = very significant
M = moderately significant
NV = not very significant

As you probably already know, negative cues can be pretty hard to overcome. The idea, then, is to create positive cues that remind you to do more activity throughout the day. Some positive cues include:

- placing exercise clothing or walking shoes where you can see them
- having a friend or your spouse call just before your activity time
- writing yourself notes as reminders
- hanging the dog's leash on the doorknob.

At the same time, remove as many negative cues as possible. If you're a TV addict, hide the remote or unplug the set; if you usually read the paper when you get home, wait to buy it until after you have accomplished your daily activity goal.

Plan for the unexpected

Life is full of surprises. Even when you have every intention of meeting your activity goals, challenges can arise. Occasional breaks in an activity routine are sometimes unavoidable. Vacation or business travel, times when your work or your family demands more of your time, periods of bad weather, and an illness or injury are challenges that face most of us from time to time. When you come to these bumps in the road, the decision to take a positive approach is critical to your success.

One helpful way to avoid getting off track is to plan ahead. Before challenging situations occur, create an "emergency plan." You may have to be flexible about the time of day you do your activity, for example. Or you may have to re-evaluate your activity goals and set them at a more achievable level for a while. Even if you do less than your usual amount of activity, remember that doing something is always better than doing nothing. And be sure to keep your self-talk positive during trying times. Avoid "all-

or-nothing" thinking and feelings of failure. Sometimes it's necessary to remind yourself "I'm doing the best I can."

Self-monitoring and record keeping

As part of your diabetes care plan, you're probably already keeping records of your blood glucose test results, the foods you eat, and how much and what types of medication you take (if not, you should be!). So you know that while record keeping takes some time and commitment, it has many advantages. In other words, the benefits far outweigh the costs. Adding an activity log to your records also has benefits, since the information you collect can help you make decisions about how to achieve your activity goals. An activity log can:

- measure your daily successes and challenges
- track your progress toward achieving long-term activity goals
- increase your awareness of your activity-related thoughts and feelings
- increase your feelings of satisfaction and enjoyment related to doing activity
- prevent relapse by helping to identify sticking points and early signs of a drop-off in activity
- aid with troubleshooting by helping to identify alternative or better ways of fitting activity into your lifestyle

Figure 2-2 shows a sample activity log form. Since keeping a log should also be fun and easy, feel free to modify the form to suit your needs. As long as the log provides feedback about your progress and helps you create a lasting activity habit, it can be as simple or as detailed as you want.

Are you ready to go?

Changing your lifestyle is rarely easy, but using strategies such as setting goals, making a contract, practicing positive self-talk, and creating an activity log will help you get there. You may find that some of these strategies work for you while others don't. Just remember to be positive and open-minded.

Figure 2-2 Sample Activity Record

Activity Record

	SUN.	MON.	TUES.	WED.	THURS.	FRI.	SAT.

Type of Activity

1._____

2._____

3._____

Amount of Time

Session 1_____

Session 2_____

Session 3_____

Enjoyment
1. Very enjoyable
2. Somewhat enjoyable
3. Neutral
4. Somewhat unenjoyable
5. Very unenjoyable

Support System

Successes/Challenges

Self-Monitoring

Blood glucose:_____

Heart rate:_____

Perceived exertion:_____

Blood pressure:_____

King, A.C., and J.E. Martin. *Resource Manual for Guidelines for Exercise Testing and Prescription*. Durstine, J.L. et al eds. The American College of Sports Medicine, 2nd ed, Philadelphia, PA: Lea and Febiger, 1993: 443-454.

3

Building an Activity Program

Achieving 30 Minutes per Day

Be physically inefficient! It may sound strange, but it's the key to fitting 30 minutes of activity into your day the easy way. All you need to do is identify good chances to do things in a physically active—but not necessarily quick or easy—way throughout the day. It can be as simple as giving up the remote control so that you have to get out of your chair and walk over to the TV to turn it on or off. By being more physically inefficient you can fit activity into your daily routine, no matter how busy you are. By doing 30 minutes of moderate activity on most days of the week, you can burn an extra 150 calories per day or about 1,000 calories per week—a level of calorie burning that can result in health benefits. If you have not been doing any activity at all, simply start by doing something, no matter how little, and gradually build up from there.

Get Your Muscles Moving

The large muscles of the body include the leg, arm, shoulder, and back muscles. When you do activities like walking, mowing the lawn, swimming, stair climbing, biking, or vacuuming, you use large muscles in a repetitive and continuous way. These types of activities can improve your health in a variety of ways. They:

- strengthen the large muscles themselves
- strengthen the heart muscle
- improve the body's ability to use oxygen efficiently
- promote calorie burning, weight loss, and loss of body fat
- help reduce blood glucose levels
- improve stamina, endurance, and energy level

Because these activities offer many important benefits and are quite easy to fit into your daily routine, finding ways to do a few short sessions each day can be a good way to increase your level of activity. Here are a few ideas:

- walk more whenever possible
- park your car farther away when shopping or at work
- instead of putting your dog out in the yard, walk him down the street
- if you use public transportation, get off a stop or two early and walk the added distance
- take your children or grandchildren out for a walk as part of the day's activities
- schedule short walking breaks each hour and walk around your office or home for a few minutes
- if a destination is within walking distance, put away the car keys and walk instead
- walk or march in place while watching TV or talking on the phone
- give up remote controls and other energy-saving devices that prevent you from getting up and walking even a short distance
- take a walk just for the fun of it
- take the stairs instead of the elevator for at least one floor. If climbing is difficult for you, start off by just walking down
- do your own yard work
- do your own housekeeping
- if you have a stationary bicycle, ride it while you read the paper or watch TV
- choose hobbies like golf, gardening, swimming, walking, tennis, and dancing instead of watching TV, going to the movies, or playing computer games

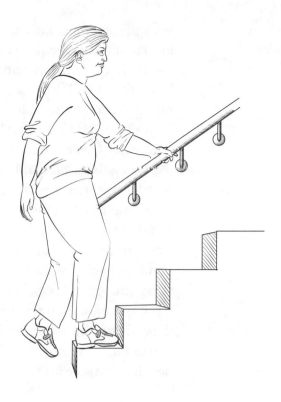

Don't overdo it!   These activities should feel energizing, but they should not feel hard to do at all. There are a couple of ways to tell if you are doing enough physical activity without pushing yourself too hard. The easiest way is to do the "talk test." You should always be able to talk to someone while you are doing an activity. If you become so short of breath that you can't talk, you should slow down. Why? First, if the activity feels uncomfortable or difficult, you are less likely to stick with it. Second, if you do too much too fast, you may become tired or injured. So remember, be kind and gentle with yourself. This is especially important when you are just beginning to increase activity in your daily routine.

The other way of determining if you are exercising at a comfortable rate is to rely on your own viewpoint of how difficult the activity feels. A guideline called the Borg RPE (Rating of Perceived Exertion) Scale was developed as a simple method of rating how much effort you feel an activity requires while you are doing it. Many factors can influence your perception of how an activity feels. These include your level of fitness, whether you are well-rested when you begin the activity, and environmental variables like heat and humidity. The RPE scale considers all these factors. The ratings listed on the scale are related to how hard your heart is working and to how well your body uses oxygen during an activity (see Figure 3-1).

Using this scale can help you do an activity at an enjoyable level without working yourself to the point that you'll never want to exercise again. When you do an activity, you shouldn't expect to feel 0 on the scale, or "nothing at all." You want to feel a bit more challenged than that. On the other hand, the activity should not feel in the range of 7 to 10—"very strong" or "very, very strong/maximal"—either. That is too much effort and will probably be very uncomfortable. If the activity feels in the range of 3 to 5 on the Borg scale, or "moderate" to "strong," you are gaining health and fitness benefits from the activity without pushing yourself too hard.

Figure 3-1 Borg Rating of Perceived Exertion (RPE) Scale

0	Nothing at all
0.5	Very, very weak
1	Very Weak
2	Weak
3	Moderate
4	Somewhat strong
5	Strong
6	
7	Very strong
8	
9	
10	Very, very strong
	Maximal

From: Borg GA. Physiologic basis of physical exertion. *Med Sci Sports Exerc.* 1982; 14: 377–387.
Hanson P. Clinical exercise testing. In: Blair SN et al eds. *The American College of Sports Medicine Resource Manual for Guidelines for Exercise Testing and Prescription.* Philadelphia, PA: Lea & Febiger; 1998: 213–214.

Push, Pull, and Lift

All of your body's muscles, even small ones, benefit from being called upon to do some work. Activities that require pushing, pulling, and lifting—or resistance activities—can help strengthen specific muscles or groups of muscles. Make it a point to include resistance activities in your day. They:

- increase muscle strength
- improve muscle tone
- help reduce risk of osteoporosis and bone fractures
- help improve balance and reduce risk of falls
- increase muscle mass and help with weight control
- increase energy level and improve fitness
- increase the body's sensitivity to insulin

Examples of resistance activities include light weight lifting, moderate calisthenics, and strengthening exercises that use elastic bands for resistance. You do not have to purchase special equipment to do these activities unless you wish to; you probably have a set of weights already! You can use household items like canned foods, thick books, or certain types of tools as weights. But don't be concerned about that yet. Simply lifting the weight of an arm or leg against the pull of gravity can work your muscles, so you may not need any extra resistance at first. Later, as you gain strength, you can experiment with simple "equipment" to make pulling, pushing, or lifting more challenging. You can do many strengthening activities even while sitting in a chair (page 95), so try them while you watch TV, talk on the phone, or take a break at your desk during the workday.

In going about many of our routine daily tasks, most of us already do pushing, pulling, and lifting activities. Some examples of resistance activities from your daily routine include:

Lifting
- carrying a briefcase into your office
- bringing a load of groceries into your house
- taking the day's trash outside

Pushing
- mowing your lawn
- pushing a child in a stroller

Pulling
- weeding your garden
- rolling a suitcase on wheels through an airport

In addition to helping you complete your daily chores, all of these activities help strengthen muscles. So don't shy away from doing them!

Of course, how you push, pull, and lift is very important. Doing too much of an activity, doing too many of these activities, or doing them in the wrong way can lead to injury—and with injured muscles, it's hard to get any exercise at all! To perform physical activities in a safe manner, remember to:

- keep it comfortable
- start slowly and gradually build up

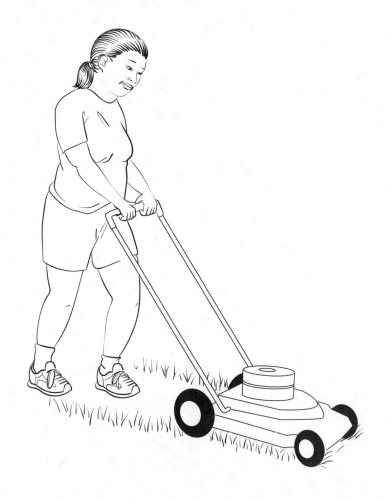

- do slow, steady, controlled movements
- avoid jerking or straining
- position your body properly
- focus on breathing (don't hold your breath!)
- cut back if you feel pain, soreness, or stiffness

Stretch and Relax

Stretching is an effective activity that is very simple to do, requires little pre-planning, and doesn't require any special equipment. In fact, some formal activity programs, like yoga, are nothing more than stretching. It is an activity that you can do nearly any time and almost anywhere. Take a few mini-breaks throughout the day to do a few stretches, and soon you will feel more energized and more relaxed. Before you know it, you will be looking for any opportunity to stretch!

As an important part of a well-balanced activity routine, stretching benefits your body in several important ways. It:

- increases flexibility
- increases range of motion of joints
- reduces stiffness
- reduces risk of muscle and joint injury
- reduces risk of developing back pain
- relieves muscular tension and pain

Like any exercise, there is a right way and a wrong way to stretch. Stretching should always feel mild and relaxing; it should never feel uncomfortable and painful. Here are some do's and don'ts of stretching.

Do:
- relax as you stretch
- stretch only to the point that you feel mild tension
- hold a steady stretch for 5 to 15 seconds
- breathe deeply and slowly
- keep it comfortable
- ease off the stretch if you feel discomfort

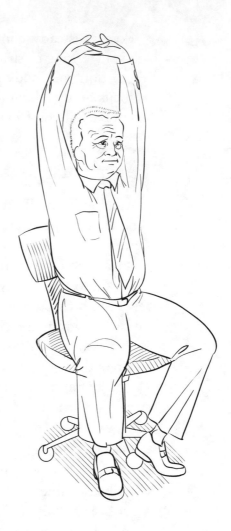

Don't:
- bounce or bob
- focus on tension-creating thoughts
- hold your breath
- strain or push to the point of pain

How long should each activity session last?

It's up to you to decide how long an activity session lasts. Of course, many factors can influence the amount of time you spend doing an activity, such as time limitations, your level of fitness and conditioning, and how difficult the activity is for you to do. For example, you may be able to walk comfortably for 10 minutes and have time to do this during your lunch break. However, if you decide to climb the stairs to your office in the morning you may find that one flight is the most you can do at first. Or you may be rushed for time in the morning and decide to squeeze activity into a shorter session for this reason. As you gain fitness and skill at juggling activity time, you may decide to increase the length of either session.

Remember to look for opportunities to do things in an active way throughout the day. You can, at any time, benefit from doing a brief session of stretching or light calisthenics—even without getting up out of your chair. Short sessions add up, and each one contributes to a daily activity total.

Be active all day! Squeeze as many activity sessions into a day as you can do comfortably. Remember, the ultimate goal is to build up to doing 30 minutes of activity per day for improved health. One way to do this is to simply do things in a more energy inefficient way. Look for ways to make small changes in your routine so that you gradually build in more physical activity. Cut back on the amount of time you spend doing "inactivities" like sitting for a long period of time. Get up and move often. Take frequent mini-breaks to do some stretching, easy pushing, pulling and lifting activities, or a few minutes of walking.

Another option is to do fewer activity sessions but to have each one last longer. You can do just one, two, or maybe three sessions per day and have each one last for between 10 and 30 minutes. For example, on weekends, you may enjoy sharing activity time with a friend and decide to walk together for 30 minutes then do some stretching afterward. In this case, you are able to accomplish your daily activity goal in just one session. During the week you may choose to do three shorter activity sessions. If you walk your dog for 10 minutes in the morning, for example, then take a 10-minute walk during lunch, and do 15 minutes of stretching and strengthening activities in the evening, you've accomplished 35 minutes of activity. Just how you accumulate activity time throughout the day is up to you. You can either do short sessions frequently or longer sessions less frequently. The most important thing is to be creative and flexible in finding ways to achieve your activity goals.

Building on your exercise foundation

Now you have the material that you need to start building a daily activity routine that you find fun and energizing. Remember, there are three types of activities that are the foundation of any well-planned daily routine:

- large muscle movement activities
- pulling, pushing, and lifting activities
- stretching activities

With these building blocks in hand, your first task is to look at each day and figure out how to best fit in an activity at any given time. For example, if you have the option of walking down the street to visit a neighbor or driving your car, take the active option. Use your large muscles and walk. If you have the choice of pushing your own cart out of the grocery store and loading your groceries into your car or of having someone do it for you, take the active option and do the pushing and lifting yourself. It is a great opportunity to keep muscles strong without taking up a lot of time. When you watch TV at night, you can either sit passively or you can do some stretching while you watch. Do the stretching. It will feel great and it will not cost any additional free time.

Each of these types of activities can fit into your routine in a unique way just as each type offers its own special set of benefits. The following chapter presents specific ideas on how you can fit physical activity into each day. Draw upon these ideas, experiment and try them out so that you can become physically active in a way that you enjoy.

4 Be Active Everywhere

Most of our daily life is spent in three places: at home, work, and out in the community. Fortunately, all three settings offer lots of opportunities for doing physical activity. At home, light exercise can be worked into housework, yard work, and family time; at the office, a short activity break can be a welcome relief from the day's stress; and out in the community, exercise can be mixed into running errands or going out for entertainment. With just a little bit of planning, including daily activity "in" these three areas of your life can add up to a fun and easy fitness routine.

Getting the Most Out of Every Activity

You may not know it, but you can reap physical gains from doing even the simplest task. The trick is to focus on doing it in an active and vigorous way. For example, when you mow the lawn or vacuum the floor, pick up the pace a little bit to give your heart a better workout. Actively push and pull with your arms and shoulders so that they benefit and get stronger from the work. When you unload the clothes dryer or prepare to hang laundry out on the line, bend your knees a little more than usual as you pick up the items. This will help strengthen your leg muscles. And as you hang clothes on the clothesline, reach and stretch a little farther than usual. This will help increase upper body strength and flexibility. Almost any task can be beneficial if you go about it in an active and vigorous manner.

If you're not quite clear on what doing things in a more "active and vigorous way" means, here is a quick demonstration: Hold your arms down at your sides so that they are relaxed and limp. Then, keeping them in this fairly floppy state, lift them out to the side, then up over your head and back down to your sides. How did the activity feel? Probably it didn't feel like much work for your muscles. Now, hold your arms down at your sides again, only this time tense the muscles in your arms and shoulders and point your fingers down to the floor. Maintaining this tension, slowly lift your arms up. (Think about stretching and reaching for the walls as you lift your arms to the side then overhead toward the ceiling.) Take a deep breath in as you reach up. Then maintaining this tension and energy, return your arms to the starting position, breathing out as you do this. How did the activity feel this time? Did you feel your muscles do work? Did you feel a good stretch? Did you feel invigorated as you breathed in deeply and then exhaled? The answer is probably, Yes! That is the benefit of doing even routine tasks in an active and vigorous way.

Being Active at Home

There is no place like home, especially if you are looking to become more physically active. Your home offers the most options for fitting activity into your day. Each work-related task or leisure activity you do has the potential to benefit you in a variety of ways. For example, if you enjoy baking bread (without help from a bread machine), you can give your arms, shoulders, and back a good workout—especially if you vigorously push, pull, and lift as you knead the dough. You also work in a bit of stretching. If you decide to go for a walk in the evening, you will gain very different benefits: Walking uses large muscles in your legs, and exercises your heart muscle as well. But unlike kneading bread, walking doesn't give your upper body much work to do. So walking and baking bread each offer unique benefits in terms of which muscles they use and how they use them. A key point to remember is that if you do both activities in a day, you get all the benefits! That is why doing a variety of daily activities, both at work and at play, is so desirable.

To take this example one step farther, baking bread and walking also differ in the number of calories you burn while doing them. Table 4-1 looks at chores that most of us do at home, the average number of calories burned in 30 minutes, and the types of activity benefits the chores offer (large muscle movement, stretching, or push, pull, and lift). Cooking and baking are considered "light" activities when it comes to calorie burning; they burn 90 to 100 calories in 30 minutes. Walking is a "moderate" activity; when you walk for 30 minutes, you burn about 150 calories. Examples of a

Table 4-1 Activity Benefits of Household Chores and Yard Work

ACTIVITY CATEGORY	AVERAGE CALORIES BURNED/ 30 MINUTES*	TYPE OF ACTIVITY BENEFITS
Light Household Chores	90 to 100 calories	
Cooking/baking		PPL, STR
Dusting furniture		STR
Laundry		PPL, STR
Light carpentry		PPL, STR
Sweeping floors		LMM, STR
Washing dishes		PPL
Moderate House and Yard Work	130 to 190 calories	
Gardening		LMM, PPL, STR
Mowing the lawn/hedging and trimming		LMM, PPL
Raking leaves		LMM, PPL, STR
Scrubbing floors		LMM, PPL, STR
Carrying out trash or recycling		LMM, PPL
Vacuuming floors		LMM, PPL, STR
Washing cars		LMM, PPL, STR
Washing windows		LMM, PPL, STR
Hard House and Yard Work	over 200 calories	
Digging light earth		LMM, PPL
Shoveling snow		LMM, PPL
Home repair		LMM

Key: LMM = large muscle movement; PPL = push, pull, lift; STR = stretch.
 *Calories burned per 30 min are determined for an individual who weighs 150 pounds. Actual calories burned are slightly less for individuals who weigh under 150 pounds and are slightly more for individuals who weigh over 150 pounds. It is assumed that activities are done with moderate effort.

"hard" activity—one that requires more effort to complete and burns 200 calories or more in 30 minutes—would be shoveling snow, digging in the garden, or doing home repair.

The tasks of everyday living are not always fun or rewarding, so it is nice to know that when you do physical work around the house or in the yard it can at least contribute significantly to your overall health. As you study Table 4-1, notice that many tasks offer more than one activity benefit, increasing their contributions to your health and fitness.

Being active at play

Leisure time at home is valuable time that we should all budget for, even during the busiest periods in our lives. It's our opportunity to do things simply for enjoyment. And if your leisure time is physically active, it has the added benefit of contributing to your good health and fitness. Table 4-2 identifies a variety of leisure activities, their calorie-burning potential, and the types of activity benefits they offer. Like work-related tasks, each leisure activity offers a unique set of benefits, and can contribute to overall fitness in more than one way.

Notice that very light leisure activities require little movement, so the calories you burn and the activity benefits you gain from them are pretty small. You should limit the amount of time you spend doing these "inactivities." If you enjoy reading or watching TV, consider riding a stationary bicycle, walking on a treadmill, or marching in place at the same time. This way you can turn inactive leisure time into activity time. But even if you're just sitting back watching TV, you can be active. On page p. 95 you'll find a series of stretching and strengthening activities to do while you sit in an armchair. By practicing the exercises, you can gain flexibility, increase strength and muscle tone, and rev up calorie burning, even while you watch your favorite program. At the very least, make it a practice to avoid sitting for a long period of time. Get up every half-hour or so and take a 5-minute walk around your house, stretch for a few minutes, or do some light lifting and strengthening activities. These short activity breaks add up, and can con-

Table 4-2 Activity Benefits of Leisure Time Activities at Home

ACTIVITY CATEGORY	AVERAGE CALORIES BURNED/ 30 MINUTES*	TYPE OF ACTIVITY BENEFITS
Very Light Leisure	50 to 90 calories	
Computer games etc.		
Playing cards		
Reading		
Sewing/knitting		
Watching TV		
Light Leisure Activities	90 to 120 calories	
Billiards		STR
Bowling		PPL, STR
Stationary cycling (5 mi/hr)		LMM
Golf (riding cart)		PPL, STR
Stretching		STR
Walking/strolling (2 mi/hr)		LMM
Woodworking		PPL, STR
Moderate Leisure Activities	120 to 190 calories	
Badminton		LMM, STR
Calisthenics		PPL, STR
Cycling (8-10 mi/hr)		LMM, PPL
Dance (ballroom)		LMM, PPL, STR
Fishing (walking and wading)		LMM, PPL, STR
Golf (walking and carrying clubs)		LMM, PPL, STR
Table tennis		LMM, STR,
Tennis (recreational)		LMM, PPL, STR
Volleyball		LMM, PPL, STR
Water exercise (aerobics)		LMM, PPL, STR
Walking (3 mi/hr)		LMM
Hard Leisure Activities	200 or more calories	
Cycling (> 10 mi/hr)		LMM, PPL
Vigorous dance (aerobic, square dance)		LMM, PPL, STR
Handball		LMM, PPL
Jogging (> 5 mi/hr)		LMM
Swimming (Moderate effort)		LMM, PPL, STR
Tennis (competitive)		LMM, PPL, STR
Brisk walking (> 4 mi/hr)		LMM
Weight lifting (vigorous effort)		PPL

Key: LMM = large muscle movement; PPL = push, pull, lift; STR = stretch.

*Calories burned per 30 min are determined for an individual who weighs 150 pounds. Actual calories burned are slightly less for individuals who weigh under 150 pounds and are slightly more for individuals who weigh over 150 pounds. It is assumed that activities are done with moderate effort.

tribute significantly to your activity goals and improved health.

If you build some moderate activity into your leisure time, you see both health benefits and calorie-burning potential increase. That is why the Surgeon General suggests accumulating 30 minutes of moderate intensity physical activity each day. A commitment to doing moderate activity may lead you to try new, fun forms of recreation or to resume leisure activities that you may have enjoyed in the past but haven't done recently.

Here are some fun ways to fit moderate activity into your day:

- take a walk or hike with family or friends. You can do this in your neighborhood or go to a park for a special outing
- take your children (or grandchildren) to a neighborhood playground or outside in the yard and play!
- play a backyard game of badminton, volleyball, or croquet
- play catch or shoot some baskets
- play some favorite music and dance (children love this too)
- if you have a backyard or neighborhood pool, get in and enjoy playing and moving in the water
- learn something new like yoga or aerobic dance by plugging a tape into your VCR (you can rent tapes from your local movie rental store)

If you are used to doing vigorous exercise, moderate activities may be too easy for you. However, before you attempt "hard" leisure activities, it is important to have a complete medical examination by your physician. More vigorous activities offer the advantage of burning more calories, but they also carry a greater risk of exercise-related injury than do moderate activities. This is especially true if you try to do "hard" activities before you are physically ready. It is very important to start slowly and—as you become more fit—gradually increase exercise intensity.

Getting the Most from Your Walk

You can get health benefits by walking at any speed. But if you're looking for greater fitness gains—weight loss, stronger muscles, increased heart/lung stamina—experts have a few tips. As always, check with your physician before beginning or making a change in your fitness program.

- Make it brisk. A leisurely stroll will help relax and energize you, but a brisk walk—3 to 4 miles per hour—will give your heart a good workout and burn more calories. Just be sure to walk at a pace that allows you to pass the "talk test."
- Take more steps. If you want to speed up your walk, don't lengthen your stride. That can feel awkward and also cause pain in your knees, shins, and feet. Instead, step more quickly, all the while maintaining a comfortable, natural stride.
- Pump your arms. Swinging your arms down by your sides as you walk can cause discomfort in the back. Instead bend your elbows, hold them close to your body at waist level, and pump them back and forth as you walk. This will help you go faster and will avoid stress on your lower back.

On the town   Another way to work activity into your leisure time is to make it part of everything you do when you're out on the town. For instance:

- Look for ways to build activity into inactive entertainment.
- When you go to movies, arrive early to buy your tickets, then walk until it's time to go in for the show.
- If you are out shopping for pleasure, budget time to do some extra walking and window shopping.

- Find out about walking programs at your favorite mall. Plan your leisure-time shopping trips so that they match up with times when you can join other "mall walkers" in doing some uninterrupted, brisk walking before you shop.
- When you dine out, take advantage of opportunities to window shop or stroll in a park or along a waterfront area either while you wait to be seated, or after you have finished your meal.
- If a restaurant is within walking distance of your home, don't touch those car keys! Make walking your mode of transportation.
- Avoid using valet parking. As long as it is safe to do so, park your own car and walk to restaurants and other establishments that offer valet parking.
- When you go to concerts, the theater, or other performances, arrive early and take a short walk to explore the area around the theater before the program begins. Always get up to stretch and walk during intermissions.
- Plan special, active outings with family and friends at parks or recreation areas.
- Try out recreational activities that you may have enjoyed in the past, such as bowling or miniature golf.
- Consider trying ballroom, country, or other types of dance. Dancing can be a fun and vigorous way to increase activity during an evening out.
- Play golf on courses where you are allowed to walk and carry or pull your clubs.
- Go to a driving range or to batting cages where you can challenge yourself, sharpen your skills, and get some exercise at the same time.
- Join a non-competitive tennis league.
- Take a class to learn yoga, tai chi, water aerobics, or other non-competitive forms of exercise and movement.
- Learn about popular areas for walking, cycling, or cross-country skiing in your city and try them out. Many cities have developed path or walkway systems where people can enjoy these activities in safe, park-like settings.
- Join a walking, cycling, or swimming club.

- Go fishing and walk or hike between fishing holes.
- Do active volunteer work that you enjoy. Hospitals, youth programs, schools, museums, zoos, parks, and environmental associations often need and value the support of volunteers.

Leisure activities can take as much or as little time as you wish. Make it your goal to substitute "inactivities" with active leisure time. A good way to start is to keep track of how much time you spend sitting and being inactive during your free time each day. Then choose enjoyable, active alternatives to fill that time (Figure 4-1). In this way, you don't have to make time for activity; you can simply put the time you have to active, healthy use.

Being Active on the Job

Even in this age of economy, efficiency, and labor-saving devices in the work place, most American workers feel very pressed for time. Between long commutes and other demands that extend the workday, personal time is shrinking. And worse, the typical day at work has become so inactive that it actually can be harmful to one's health. In fact, a number of studies completed over the past 40 years have shown that people who are inactive at work have higher death rates than do people who work in physically active jobs. Studies have also associated physical inactivity with a substantial number of deaths due to type 2 diabetes and related complications. So, it is important to examine your typical workday and look at how active or inactive it is.

Table 4-3 offers examples of some physically active and some physically inactive jobs. Notice that the active jobs require people to do a fair amount of walking, as well as some pushing, pulling, and lifting. The inactive jobs involve a lot of sitting and very little movement. If your work requires you to do a lot of sitting or to be very inactive for long periods of time, it is especially important for you to find ways to build activity breaks into your day. However, even if your job is fairly physically active, you can benefit from

Figure 4-1 Home Activity Evaluation

	TYPE OF ACTIVITY		
	INACTIVE	ACTIVE ALTERNATIVE	
	SITTING/LYING DOWN	WORK	LEISURE
Morning			
7:00-8:00			
8:00-9:00			
9:00-10:00			
10:00-11:00			
11:00-12:00			
Afternoon			
12:00-1:00			
1:00-2:00			
2:00-3:00			
3:00-4:00			
4:00-5:00			
5:00-6:00			
Evening			
6:00-7:00			
7:00-8:00			
8:00-9:00			
9:00-10:00			
10:00-11:00			

Night time sleep from _____ to _____

activity breaks to do some stretching and relieve muscle tension.

How to increase activity at work

Let's look at how you can build activity into your workday without taking time away from your actual duties. First and foremost, find opportunities to do small amounts of activity often throughout the day. This basic principle will help you to easily and successfully become more active at work. Here are some specific examples of ways to squeeze activity into your workday:

- Get up 10 minutes or 15 minutes earlier than usual and spend this time doing some activity before work. Take your dog for a walk or spend the extra minutes walking on the way into your office. Or do some stretching and light calisthenics after your morning shower, such as the Stretch and Strengthen Routine in Chapter 7.
- If you're in the habit of grabbing a fast food meal on your commute, don't use the drive-through window: Park your car and walk into the restaurant—and always make the healthiest possible food choices!
- If safe to do so, park your car at a distant part of the office parking lot so that you can increase the amount of walking you do on your way in.
- If you use public transportation, get off a stop or two early and walk to your final destination.
- Use stairs instead of the elevator. If need be, take the elevator part of the way and the stairs the rest of the way, then gradually increase the number of floors you climb as you become more fit.

Table 4-3 Examples of Physically Active vs. Physically Inactive Jobs

PHYSICALLY ACTIVE JOBS	PHYSICALLY INACTIVE JOBS
Carpenter/painter	Bank teller
Chef	Clerical worker
Farmer	Computer programmer
House cleaner	Driver (bus, cab, truck etc.)
Landscape/yard worker	Musician
Machinist	Sales
Nurse	Telemarketer
Steel mill/heavy industrial worker	Writer
Store clerk	
Tailor	
Teacher	
Waitress	

- If you go out for lunch, walk to your destination.
- Before you begin your commute home, take a walk. You may manage to miss the traffic rush and still get home at the usual time.
- When you have to work at your desk for an extended period of time, build short breaks into your day. For example:
  - Do a series of seated stretches (see page 95)
  - Do a few easy pulling, pushing, or lifting activities at your desk (see page 95)
  - Get up and take a quick walk around your office or go to the water fountain, mail drop, or copy machine
  - Use a speakerphone or a mobile phone so that you can get up and pace around your office during phone calls. If you don't have these options, stand up or do some chair exercises (page 95) during phone calls
  - Eat lunch at your desk, then walk during your lunch break

As you can see, these suggestions require very little time, and you can do many of them while you work. For example, do foot and toe stretches while you are at your computer or a few seated knee extensions while you sit in a meeting. And those short activity sessions that allow you to leave your work for a few minutes can be very beneficial and are usually well justified, too. When you return you will be re-energized, more focused, more productive, and less tense than before the activity session.

It is not necessary to have special exercise equipment at work to successfully increase daily activity. However, if you plan to take short walks or climb stairs as part of your fitness routine, it is important to wear comfortable and supportive shoes. If you plan to take fairly long walks during lunch or after work, keep a good pair of walking shoes and athletic socks in your office so that you can change into them for the activity. This will make sure you're comfortable and will minimize the risk of injury to your feet from ill-fitting shoes—an important consideration if you have neuropathy. You may also decide to keep an exercise band or a pair of light weights in your desk drawer; you can use them to add effort to pushing, pulling, or lifting activities that you do at your desk. A can of soda or a book can serve nicely as a dumb bell for increasing resistance as well.

As always, the overall goal is to keep it simple and do small amounts of activity frequently throughout the workday. If you do just two minutes of activity each hour during an eight-hour workday and walk for 20 minutes during your lunch break, you will accumulate 36 minutes of physical activity—enough to significantly improve your health!

On the road   Work-related travel can really disrupt your exercise routine, but luckily, there are ways to meet the challenge. Once again the basic principle of doing small amounts of activity frequently throughout the day will help you stay physically active when you're on the road. Here are some suggestions for fitting in activity on travel days:

- When you travel by air:
  - budget time to walk to your flight instead of using shuttles, trains, or moving walkways in airports
  - if you have a carry-on bag, even one on wheels, think about actively using your arm, shoulder, and back muscles as you pull, push, and lift it on your way through the airport
  - do some stretches on the airplane or while you wait for your flight. See the seated stretches on page 95
  - during a long flight, get up and move periodically. If you can find some space at the back of the plane, do some standing stretches (see page 105)
- When you travel by car:
  - make time to get out of your car every few hours and walk for five or 10 minutes
  - stretch for a few minutes whenever you stop to buy gas or make a phone call
  - when you stop for meals, always get out of your car; walk for 10 minutes either before or after you eat
- When you stay out of town:

- take advantage of down time to do some stretching and strengthening activities in your hotel room (see page 95); if you wish, pack light weights or an exercise band to use in your fitness routine
- march in place while you watch TV or turn on some music and dance
- if your hotel has an exercise facility, try it out (for example, walk on a treadmill or ride a stationary bike while you watch the evening news). If it has a pool, swim, walk, or do exercises in the water
- if safe to do so, walk and explore the city you are visiting on foot; walk to meetings or to nearby restaurants

It's true that travel can be unpredictable and tiring. As a result, your focus may simply be on getting to your destination and home again, rather than on keeping up with your daily activities. But if you create a healthy travel plan and have it in place before you leave on your trip, this will help you stay on track with activity as well as other health goals. And if you exercise, you may find it makes travel less tiring and more enjoyable. As part of your travel plan, try to identify:

- strategies for fitting small amounts of activity into your day to total at least 30 minutes. Remind yourself that even when you feel fatigued moderate physical activity can energize you
- healthy eating strategies. Don't be a victim of unhealthy, overpriced meals and snacks in airports or on the road. Remember that the availability of food on flights can be pretty unpredictable, so the best option is to bring along your own meals and snacks
- methods to ensure that you drink plenty of fluids (for example, bring along a water bottle)
- the diabetes supplies that you need to have with you (meter, strips, medications, and a treatment for hypoglycemia)

When you take steps to stay active and healthy when you travel, you will feel good, will be able to enjoy your travels, and will be focused and productive when working.

Really Run Those Errands!

Most Americans spend a lot of time out-and-about around town running errands, doing household shopping, or going to appointments. Unfortunately, because of suburban sprawl, we are likely to spend more time driving and parking our cars than burning calories doing our chores. Few of us have the option of running errands in a neighborhood or tightly spaced downtown area as we did in the past, so we need to find ways to build activity back into our lives when we are out-and-about.

Fitting it all in

You probably feel rushed when you're out running errands or taking care of appointments and other personal business. But with some planning ahead and willingness to change your usual habits, it is possible to fit in quick activity sessions during these times. The benefit is noticeably higher activity levels, improved health, and reduced feelings of stress, strain, and fatigue when you return home.

So, let's consider strategies for building activity into the routine task of running errands and taking care of personal business.

- Have your trip planned and organized before you start out.
  - Determine the most efficient route for driving in order to minimize the amount of time you spend sitting in your car.
  - If possible, schedule appointments and run errands when you know that traffic and crowds are the lightest. This will help prevent a sense of urgency, which can be a big barrier to fitting in activity.
  - Organize your trip so that you cluster errands together if they are near each other. Then park your car once and walk between stops.
- Make an effort to walk whenever possible.

- If safe to do so, park your car at the far end of parking lots so that you increase the amount of walking you do on your way into stores and businesses.
- Walk between errands when the stores and businesses you need to visit are close to one another.
- If you have errands to do at a mall, schedule your day so that you do them in the morning. Then arrive 30 minutes before the stores open and join the mall walkers in doing some brisk walking before you start shopping.
- Take stairs instead of escalators and elevators.
- Avoid using drive-through windows. Always get out of your car and walk into businesses that offer drive-through options, such as banks, restaurants, and dry cleaners.
- If you use public transportation, get off a stop or two away from your final destination and walk the added distance.
- Whenever you do walk, make an effort to pick up the pace a bit and walk briskly!
- Use your own muscles and "people power" to push, pull, and lift.
  - Carry your own groceries and packages.
  - Load at least some of your groceries and other packages into the car yourself.
  - When you have the option, avoid using doors that open automatically. Instead, push or pull doors open yourself.
  - If you are standing and waiting in a line, do some arm, shoulder, or neck stretches (see page 95).
  - If you are sitting and waiting, do a few chair exercises or stretches (see page 95).

You may not be able to say you literally "ran" those errands, but you certainly picked up the pace and did them in an active way! And that's the important thing to remember: If you want to make activity and improved health and fitness a part of your life forever, it can be as simple as doing everything–from housework to play to travel–in a more active way. Decide to leave the car and walk when you can. Decide to climb stairs instead of riding escalators and elevators. Decide to carry your own packages and open a door. You don't have to carry all the groceries or climb every flight; you just have to start one step–or one push, pull, or lift–at a time.

5

Keep Going
Activity for a Lifetime!

Setting Goals for a Lifetime of Physical Activity

Every New Year's Day, countless people resolve to lose weight and get in shape—and they want to do it fast! The phones in fitness centers ring off the hook, new members join, and members who haven't been there in months start to show up. The exercise classes are full and all the workout equipment is in use at peak times of the day. For a while, people exercise like crazy, but within a month or six weeks many begin to drop out and things slow down to the normal pace. Within three to six months, only half of the people who started to exercise will continue to stick with it. This same scenario plays out in weight loss or weight management centers too. The phones ring and people join programs and start dieting to lose those extra pounds fast! But before long, many dieters get tired of feeling hungry and restricted in their eating and are frustrated when they fail to shed all the weight they had hoped to lose in an impossibly short amount of time. So they quit.

These people make the mistake of looking for a quick fix rather than making a commitment to a long-term lifestyle change. Unfortunately, the end result of quick-fix thinking is typically repeated failure, frustration, and little progress toward achieving better health and fitness.

Quick-fix thinking doesn't fit with the whole idea of becoming more physically active for lifelong health and well-being. Consider this: Within two weeks of dropping out of an exercise program, health benefits begin to disappear. And within three months of dropping out, health gains from previous physical activity disappear altogether. So, it pays to think long-term about establishing a physical activity habit that will help you achieve a lifetime of great health and physical fitness.

Developing a fitness habit

Building moderate amounts of physical activity into your lifestyle is a difficult and important first step toward healthy, active living. Congratulations! Now it's time to go a step further and make a lifelong commitment. This means forming a physical activity habit. Creating such a habit is an ongoing process that involves goal setting as well as a number of other tactics. For long-term success, you'll need to:

- Continue to frequently examine and adjust your physical activity goals.
- For the first three to six months after starting to add lifestyle activity to your daily routine, reevaluate your fitness goals every two weeks and adjust them as needed.
- Keep your goals challenging and motivating, yet realistic. Remember that if they are too easy to reach, your goals may not be challenging enough to keep you motivated. If your goals are too difficult to achieve, you can become frustrated and discouraged, which can result in a sense of failure.
- At challenging times, when it is difficult to fit in activity, be flexible and try different things. Be willing to adapt and reset goals at an easier level for a while.
- Update and change the contract with yourself to reflect your changing goals.
- Every once in a while change the rewards you give yourself so that they continue to motivate you and reinforce your exercise habit.

Once you establish a firm habit of doing things in a physically active way each day, you will have built a solid fitness foundation. This will go a long way toward helping you remain physically active, even at times when life throws you a curve.

Now you are ready to take the next step: to further increase the amount of physical activity you do so that you can gain additional health benefits and a higher level of fitness.

What's the next step?

As your body begins to shape up, fitness and health experts recommend gradually increasing your activity time until you are able to do the amount suggested by the U.S. Surgeon General. This means 30 minutes of moderate-intensity physical activity on most, or preferably all, days of the week. To reach this level of activity, try adding time onto your activity sessions until you can do a minimum of 10 minutes of non-stop activity. Then work up to doing three 10-minute sessions of activity each day to total 30 minutes. Another alternative is to do fewer than three activity sessions but to have each one last for a longer amount of time. For example, you may choose to do one 30-minute or two 15-minute sessions of activity to accumulate a daily total of 30 minutes.

Finally, experts agree that it is possible to achieve an even higher level of fitness and greater health benefits by continuing to gradually increase the amount of activity you do. You may even get to a point where you'd like to add an exercise class or other form of structured exercise to your routine of moderate lifestyle activity. However, just remember you're not on a time clock—the progress you make and how quickly you make it is completely up to you and your comfort level.

Working toward higher activity goals

Once you are in the habit of doing a few minutes of moderate activity each day and you are comfortable with doing it, you are ready to start increasing the total amount of time you spend being physically active. Remember, at this level, you have two goals: to gradually work up to doing 30 minutes of moderate activity each day, and to gradually increase the length of each activity session until you are able to do 10 minutes of non-stop activity. The rate at which you increase activity time depends a lot on how you feel, but most experts recommend simply increasing the amount of moderate activity that you do by a minute or two each day.

Here is an example. Let's say that you are currently able to walk for five minutes comfortably without stopping and you do this three times a day—in the morning, at noon, and in the evening. Your goal is to gradually increase the amount of time that you walk during each of the three activity sessions. You eventually want to walk continuously for 10 minutes three times per day in order to achieve a daily total of 30 minutes of activity. So, the first thing you do is add one minute onto your morning walk time for a total of six minutes of walking during this session. You keep your mid-day and evening walks at five minutes each. If the longer morning walk goes well and you feel comfortable with the one-minute increase, you are probably ready to add another minute or two onto your total activity time. The next day you may decide to walk for six minutes during the mid-day and evening sessions as well. As a result, you will accumulate a daily total of 18 minutes of walking. That's a 20 percent increase in exercise, and that's good progress! Continue adding a minute or two onto your daily activity time as you're ready and soon you'll be exercising a total of 30 minutes or more each day.

Remember that you should never feel pain, too much discomfort, or fatigue as you increase the amount of activity you do. Avoid doing too much too fast. You don't want injuries or setbacks at this point. If you're injured, it's hard to do much exercise at all. In fact, you should talk to your doctor before you increase your physical activity, especially if you have questions or concerns about diabetes or other health-related issues and how they may be affected by such a change. Slow, steady, and sensible progress is healthy progress.

What about structured exercise?

After you become comfortable with increased levels of daily physical activity, you may be so happy about how you feel and look that you decide to add some structured exercise to your fitness routine. This step, though definitely a good move in terms of improving fitness and gaining health ben-

Table 5-1 Good Reasons to Consult Your Physician before Beginning Exercise

- You are a male over age 40
- You are a female over age 50
- You have diabetes and you are over age 35
- You have had type 2 diabetes for more than 10 years
- You have had type 1 diabetes for more than 15 years
- You have risk factors for coronary artery disease
  - High blood triglyceride level
  - High blood cholesterol level
  - Low HDL cholesterol level
- You have heart disease
- You have high blood pressure
- You take heart or blood pressure medications
- You have retinopathy or nephropathy including micro-albuminuria
- You have peripheral vascular disease
- You have autonomic neuropathy
- You have experienced chest pain or pressure, faintness, or dizziness
- You have a condition of your bones or joints like osteoporosis or arthritis that could be aggravated by exercise

American Diabetes Association. Position statement: Diabetes mellitus and exercise. *Diabetes Care.* 2000; 23 (suppl.1): S50-S54.

Chisholm DM, Collins MI, Davenport W, Gruber N, Kulak LL. The Par-Q validation report (modified version) by the British Columbia Department of Health. *British Columbia Medical Journal.* 1975; 17.

efits, is not necessary. But if you do decide to take part in structured exercise, consult your physician beforehand, especially if you will be doing new types of activity or more vigorous activity than before. This is particularly important if you have certain health conditions (see Table 5-1).

Adding structured exercise can improve your physical fitness to a degree that will allow you to do all the things you want to do in daily life—within reason, of course!—and to feel healthy and vigorous while doing them. However, before you get to this point, it might be helpful to understand what we really mean when we talk about "physical fitness." Basically, physical fitness is made up of four components. They are:

- **Cardiorespiratory Endurance.** This reflects the ability of the heart, lungs, and circulatory system to efficiently supply oxygen throughout the body. Cardiorespiratory endurance is measured by your ability to do aerobic exercise—activity that requires continuous, rhythmic use of large muscles—at a moderate-to-vigorous level (for example, to walk briskly for one mile).
- **Body Composition.** This component goes a step beyond simply stating your weight in pounds: It tells you what percentage of your body is lean muscle mass and what percentage is fat. For example, a football player may seem to be overweight when he tips the scales at 250 pounds, but because he is a trained athlete, he may be very muscular and have very little body fat. Having a high percentage of body fat, not just being overweight, increases health risk—including the risk of developing type 2 diabetes.
- **Muscular Strength and Endurance.** This reflects your ability to do a given amount of muscular work over a period of time. For example, a measure of your strength and endurance would be how many biceps curls you could do using a 5-pound weight and maintaining good form until you become fatigued.
- **Flexibility.** This component measures your ability to move your joints freely and without pain through a full range-of-motion. For example, rotating your shoulder joint a full 360 degrees without pain reflects excellent flexibility in that joint.

Depending on the type of structured exercise you do, it should allow you to maintain or to gradually improve one or more of these physical fitness components. Let's look at how to do this, using a guide called the FITT Principle.

Improve Your FITTness

The FITT Principle sets out exercise goals for adults who are trying to improve their health and physical fitness. Developed by experts in the field, the FITT Principle provides guidelines on exercise:

- **F**requency–how many times to exercise each week
- **I**ntensity–how vigorously or with how much effort to do an exercise
- **T**ime–how long to spend doing an exercise
- **T**ype–the kind of exercise to do

Using the FITT Principle as our guide, let's look at recommended exercise goals for improving each of the components of physical fitness.

Cardiorespiratory fitness

Improving cardiorespiratory fitness not only increases oxygen supply throughout the body, it can also improve risk factors for heart and circulatory diseases. To improve cardiorespiratory fitness, the FITT Principle recommends:

- Frequency–exercise three to five times per week
- Intensity–moderate. You should exercise at 55 to 65 percent of the maximal heart rate for your age group (see Table 5-2). Your RPE (rate of perceived exertion) should be in the 3–4 or 5 range (moderate-somewhat strong or strong; see Figure 3-1, page 30), and you should be able to talk while you exercise. If you are too out of breath to pass the "talk test," you need to slow down!
- Time–20 to 60 minutes of exercise completed in either one session of continuous activity or built up through several shorter sessions, each lasting a minimum of 10 minutes
- Type–aerobic activity that uses large muscle groups in a rhythmic, continuous way (see Table 5-3)

Body weight and body composition

If you have been struggling to lose a few pounds or if you have noticed an extra inch or two that you can pinch, you're not alone. Our society as a whole has been getting fatter, and this is due in part to our becoming "couch potatoes." Weight gain also has been linked with an increasing incidence of type 2 diabetes. Carrying extra pounds, especially around your mid-section, also increases the risk of developing heart disease and high blood pressure, as well as other chronic diseases. The good news is that a moderate weight loss of just 10 or 20 pounds can help reduce blood glucose

Table 5-2 Determining Target Heart Rate for Exercise

	EXAMPLE
1. Subtract your age from 220 to determine your age-predicted maximal heart rate (HRmax)	220 – 50 = 170
2. Multiply your HRmax by 55% and by 65% to determine your target heart rate zone for exercise in beats per minute HRmax x 0.55 = bottom of target zone HRmax x 0.65 = top of target zone	 170 x 0.55 = 93.5 (93) 170 x 0.65 = 110.5 (110)
3. Divide your target zone numbers (beats per minute) by 6 to determine your 10 second (sec) pulse count Bottom of target zone (6 ÷ lower 10 sec pulse count) Top of target zone (6 ÷ upper 10 sec pulse count)	 93 ÷ 6 = 15.6 (16) 110 ÷ 6 = 18.3 (18)
4. Your target heart rate range for aerobic exercise is between your bottom and top target zone numbers and is measured by 10 second pulse count	93–110 beats/min 16–18 beats/10 sec

Caution! *For exercise safety,* always see your physician before using a target heart rate range calculated by using this formula. This will assure that the range you calculate is correct for you. Certain heart conditions as well as heart and blood pressure medications can cause target heart rate ranges for exercise to differ from calculated values.

levels and improve your body's sensitivity to insulin, help reduce blood pressure, and improve cardiovascular risk factors. While careful meal planning is an important part of any weight loss program, physical activity is important, too. Exercise helps build and maintain lean muscle while it burns off extra body fat as fuel. Regular exercise also helps keep pounds off once they are lost. To improve your body weight and composition, the FITT Principle recommends:

- Frequency—exercise four to five times per week
- Intensity—moderate. You should exercise at 55 to 65 percent of the maximal heart rate for your age group (see Table 5-2). The RPE (rate of perceived exertion) should be in the 3–4 or 5 range (moderate-somewhat strong or strong; see Figure 3-1, page 30). And you should be able to talk while you exercise. If you are too out of breath to pass the "talk test," you need to slow down!

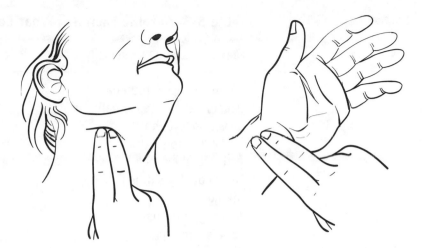

Figure 5-1: Landmarks for finding your pulse count
- using your middle and index fingers, locate your pulse at the side of your neck or base of your wrist (press down only lightly at the site)
- count the number of beats that you feel in 10 seconds—begin counting with the first beat you feel and count 0, 1, 2, 3 . . . until 10 seconds is up
- multiply your 10 second pulse count by 6 to determine your heart rate in beats per minute

- Time—30 to 60 minutes per day
- Type—aerobic activity (see Table 5-3)

When you are exercising for weight control, your main goal is to burn calories. Aim for burning about 1,000 calories per week through exercise. Experts generally agree that the safest way to reach this goal is to keep exercise intensity at a comfortable and moderate level and to exercise for the amount of time it takes to tally up 1,000 calories burned. There are a number of ways to do this:

- exercise 7 days per week and do enough activity to burn 150 calories each day
- exercise 4 days per week and do enough activity on each of those days to burn 250 calories
- exercise 3 days per week and do enough activity on each of those days to burn about 300 calories

Table 5-3 Aerobic Exercise: What Counts?

FORMS OF AEROBIC EXERCISE	CALORIES BURNED/30 MIN*
Aerobic dance/group dance[†]	205
Dance, general (e.g., ballroom)	153
Bicycling/cycling	
12-14 mph	205
Leisurely	136
Cross country skiing	272
Hiking	204
Jogging/running[†]	239
Rope skipping[†]	341
Rowing	239
Skating	239
Stair climbing[†]	204
Swimming	273
Water exercise	136
Walking	119

*Calories burned per 30 min are determined for an individual who weighs 150 pounds. Actual calories burned are slightly less for individuals who weigh under 150 pounds and are slightly more for individuals who weigh over 150 pounds. It is assumed that activities are done with moderate effort.

[†] Many of these activities are high impact. Check with your physician, especially if you have diabetes complications, to assure that these are safe options for you.

Source: Ainsworth BA, Haskell WL, Leon AS et al. Compendium of physical activities: classification of energy costs of human physical activities. *Med Sci Sports Exerc.* 1993; 25: 71-80.

The bottom line is that it is better to do long, slow, moderate exercise and be comfortable than to do hard, fast, intense activity that can be uncomfortable and can lead to muscle pain, soreness, or injury.

Muscular strength and endurance

Because we use our muscles every day to push the vacuum cleaner or lawn mower or lift a child or grandchild into our arms, it can be easy to take them for granted. When our muscles are strong we are able to work and play and do all the things we need to do each day without giving it a second thought. In the end, maintaining good muscle strength and endurance allows us to function independently and at an optimal level as we age.

The types of exercises that help keep muscles strong are called resistance or strength training activities. They include calisthenics, weight lifting, and other exercises that strengthen specific muscle groups. You don't need special equipment to do strengthening exercises. However, if you choose to use weight training equipment in a fitness center or purchase some for home use, be certain to have a trained person show you how to use the equipment safely and correctly. The strengthening exercises included in Chapter 7, in the section titled *Sit, Stretch, and Strengthen*, are some that you may wish to do at home. Follow the FITT Principle guidelines for these and other exercises to increase muscle strength and endurance. The recommendations are:

- Frequency—perform exercises two or three days per week
- Intensity—you should be able to do 12 to 15 repetitions of an exercise with good form before you become too tired. If you can easily do more repetitions than this, slightly increase the amount of weight or resistance that you work against. If you have difficulty doing this many repetitions, start with fewer repetitions (4 to 6) and gradually increase the number that you do
- Time—include eight to ten different exercises that target major muscles of the body including arm, shoulder, chest, abdominal, leg, and lower back muscles. A balanced routine usually takes 20 to 30 minutes to complete
- Type—calisthenics, weight lifting, exercise bands, or other resistance exercises

Remember these safety tips when you do resistance exercises or calisthenics:

- start slowly and gradually build up repetitions and resistance as you get stronger

- do slow, steady, and controlled movements—avoid jerking or straining
- position your body properly
- focus on breathing throughout the exercise—avoid holding your breath
- stop any exercise that causes pain—cut back if you feel soreness or stiffness
- keep it comfortable

Stretching and flexibility

Some exercisers ignore stretching and flexibility exercises because they don't seem like real exercise. However, stretching is a vital part of a balanced fitness routine. It helps you keep the ability to move your joints freely and without pain through a good range of motion. And flexible muscles are less likely to become injured. The FITT guidelines for stretching to help you achieve and maintain optimal flexibility and range of motion are:

- Frequency—perform stretches two or three days per week
- Intensity—hold a stretch just at the point where you feel mild tension
- Type—slow, steady stretching targeting major muscle groups, including arms, shoulders, chest, abdominals, lower back, and legs
- Time—hold each stretch for 10 to 30 seconds and repeat each stretch four times

When you stretch, remember these tips for comfort and safety:

- stretching should be comfortable and relaxing
- ease off if you feel pain or discomfort while stretching
- avoid bobbing, bouncing, or straining
- breathe naturally and slowly while you stretch

Putting It All Together

With these goals and guidelines in mind, let's create a formalized exercise routine. Remember, the activities that you do informally each day—including large muscle movement, pulling, pushing, lifting, and stretching—provide a solid foundation on which to build a formalized exercise routine. It is important to continue to include these unstructured activities in your day even as you introduce and then increase formalized exercise.

Before you begin to exercise, first take time to arrange the activities you plan to do into a safe and enjoyable routine. Any well-structured exercise session will include these three components:

- **Warm-up** The warm-up is intended to prepare your muscles, joints, heart, and lungs for more vigorous activity. Start with 5 to 10 minutes of light or easy aerobic activity, such as low-intensity walking or cycling, followed by 5 to 10 minutes of gentle stretching. Warm-up activities should focus on muscle groups that you plan to use during more vigorous exercise.
- **Aerobic Phase** This phase of an exercise session should include 20 to 60 minutes of aerobic activity (Table 5-3). During the aerobic phase, maintain your desired exercise intensity using target heart rate (Table 5-2), RPE (page 30), and/or the "talk test" as guides. As an option you may do three 10-minute sessions throughout the day for a total 30 minutes of aerobic exercise.
- **Cool-down** The purpose of the first part of a cool-down is to gradually bring your heart rate down to its pre-exercise level, so it should consist of 5 to 10 minutes of light or easy aerobic activity. As an alternative, follow the aerobic part of your cool-down with some easy calisthenics, weight lifting, or strengthening activities. Your cool-down should always end with some stretching.

If you choose to do strengthening exercises like weight lifting on alternate days when you don't do aerobic exercise, it is still important to include a warm-up and cool-down as part of your exercise session.

Go at your own pace

You may feel that beginning structured exercise is a step that you are ready to try now. On the other hand, you may decide that you are not ready to take this next step now or you may feel that it is well beyond your reach. Whatever your personal goals and expectations are at this point, it pays to remember the tale of the tortoise and the hare.

In this story, a fast-moving hare challenged a slow-moving tortoise to a race. At the start, the hare took off running hard and fast while the tortoise plodded along slowly and steadily. In the middle of the race, the hare decided to take a "little rest"—which became a very long rest. All the while, the tortoise kept moving along at his own pace saying to himself, "one step, another step, one step and another; slow and steady." In the end, the tortoise won the race.

When it comes to doing physical activity, whether it is informal daily activity or structured exercise, it is better to be a tortoise than a hare. Slow, steady progress leads to success. When you accept that becoming active and fit is a gradual process that takes time and commitment, you will achieve—and possibly even exceed—your own goals and

Table 5-4 Summary of Goals: Activity for Health and Exercise for Fitness

	ACTIVITY FOR HEALTH	EXERCISE FOR FITNESS
Frequency	Frequently throughout the day gradually work up to doing 10 minute sessions	3 to 5 days per week
Intensity	"Moderate"	"Moderate to vigorous" measure using heart rate = 55 to 65% age predicted maximal heart rate or RPE = 3-4-5 (moderate–somewhat strong–strong)
Time	30 minutes of daily activity	20 to 60 minutes of continuous or intermittent activity (time can be accumulated through shorter, 10 minute sessions done throughout the day)
Type	Moderate lifestyle activity/ general muscle movement	Aerobic exercise plus muscle strengthening and stretching

expectations. You will enjoy being active and fit and living vigorously. By contrast, if unrealistic goals and expectations lead you to try to do too much too fast, you will be at risk of experiencing setbacks and burnout, both of which can contribute to lack of progress and failure to succeed in the long run. So, be like the slow, steady, and consistent tortoise, not like the hare with his tendency to go hard and fast and then fizzle out. The prize at the end of the road is better health, a higher level of fitness, a greater sense of well-being, and an "I can do it" outlook.

6

Keep Your Balance
Exercise Safely with Diabetes

Hopefully by now you realize that physical activity and exercise are good for you! This is an important message to take to heart if you have diabetes or are at risk for developing the disease. Being physically active helps you manage your diabetes because exercise:

- lowers blood glucose
- improves the body's ability to use insulin
- improves cardiovascular risk factors
  - reduces high blood pressure
  - raises your HDL or "good" cholesterol level
  - reduces high triglyceride levels
- helps you lose weight or control your weight

In order to achieve these health benefits, however, you must know how to care for yourself when you exercise. Most important, you must carefully monitor your blood glucose levels.

Blood Glucose Control with Activity

The potential of physical activity to lower blood glucose levels and improve diabetes control is huge. However, a number of factors can influence the effect activity has on your blood glucose levels and you must be aware of them (See Table 6-1).

When you change your activity level or fitness routine your blood glucose may go up or down. For example, it's possible for your blood glucose to fall too low when you increase your level of activity. But if your blood glucose is poorly controlled to begin with, it can remain elevated or rise even higher with an increase in activity. In either case, managing your blood glucose can be a challenge unless you know what to do. You especially need to know what blood glucose level is considered too high, what level is too low, and what blood glucose range is just right when you exercise.

Physical activity and high blood glucose levels

First of all, it is important to establish good blood glucose control before you begin to do any activity. If your blood glucose level is too high—and especially if it has been out of control for a while—it is important to see your physician before you become more active. Your diabetes medications or meal plan may need to be adjusted to help you achieve better control. Also, it is important not to overlook other causes of high blood glucose levels, such as an infection, a cold, or the flu.

If your glucose level is high, a condition called hyperglycemia, you'll need to decide whether or not to exercise. Consider these guidelines when making your decision:

- If your blood glucose is moderately elevated due to factors such as stress or eating too much food at a meal, activity will usually have a positive blood glucose-lowering effect.
- When your blood glucose is high due to illness or infection, use common sense. It is best to wait until you feel well. Check with your physician if you have questions or concerns about your readiness to resume activity.
- If your blood glucose is 250 mg/dl or greater, it may be necessary to delay activity until you achieve better control. And remember:
- Always check your urine for ketones when your blood glucose is 250 mg/dl or higher.
- If ketones are positive, wait to exercise until your blood glucose is in a lower range and no ketones are present.
- If your blood glucose is 300 mg/dl or higher, with or without the presence of ketones, your diabetes is not under

good control. Check with your physician before beginning exercise.

High ketone levels usually occur in people with type 1 diabetes. The combination of a very high blood glucose level and ketones indicates that you don't have enough circulating insulin. And anytime you don't have enough insulin, muscles can't take in the glucose they need to meet your body's demand for extra energy during activity. When your muscles sense that they don't have enough glucose, your liver responds by increasing glucose production. In addition, your body rapidly breaks down its fat reserves for energy; ketones are byproducts of this breakdown. If ketones form faster than your body can get rid of them in urine, they build up in the blood causing it to become too acidic. As a result, blood glucose and ketone levels can continue to rise, you become dehydrated, and you are at risk for a condition called diabetic ketoacidosis (DKA). If not promptly and adequately treated, DKA can lead to coma, shock, and even death.

So, although physical activity usually helps to lower blood glucose levels, this may not be the case if your diabetes is not in good control. There are important reasons why you should see your physician and achieve better control before increasing your level of activity.

- If you exercise when your blood glucose level is over 250 mg/dl and ketones are present, you may experience an increase in glucose and ketone levels and be at risk for diabetic ketoacidosis (DKA).
- High blood glucose levels can cause you to feel tired and fatigued especially when you attempt activity. That happens because your muscles aren't supplied with the extra glucose and energy that they need for exercise. As a result, doing physical activity can feel difficult and unpleasant.
- When your blood glucose is high, you lose body fluid through repeated urination; this can cause dehydration. Doing exercise when you are dehydrated can be very stressful on your heart and cardiovascular system and can lead to poor body temperature regulation and overheating.

Physical activity alone is not a magic bullet that corrects out-of-control blood glucose levels. However, activity does contribute to better overall health and to improved long-term blood glucose control, especially when it is incorporated into a good diabetes management plan. Healthy meal planning, blood glucose monitoring, and communicating with your physician to assure that diabetes medications are appropriately adjusted are also essential.

Physical activity and low blood glucose levels

In certain situations, blood glucose levels can fall too low with activity. This is called hypoglycemia. However, not everyone who has diabetes is at risk of having this happen. A low blood glucose level is indicated by a glucose reading of 70 mg/dl or less on your meter and/or the presence of symptoms (see Table 6-1).

If you have type 2 diabetes and you are not taking certain types of diabetes pills or insulin, you are not at any greater risk of experiencing hypoglycemia with activity than someone who doesn't have diabetes. Physical activity should lead to a gradual and beneficial lowering of your blood glucose level and should help you maintain your glucose in a desirable range. So use this to your advantage!

- *A key point to remember*: Because you are not likely to experience activity-related hypoglycemia, you don't need to eat extra food when you do physical activity. Extra food can prevent you from benefiting from the blood glu-

Table 6-1 Factors that Influence the Effect of Activity on Blood Glucose Levels

- Overall diabetes control
- Blood glucose level before exercise which is influenced by:
  - Diabetes medications
  - Time of day of exercise
  - Time of exercise in relation to last meal or snack
  - Psychological factors like stress
  - Level of fitness
  - How long an activity session lasts
  - How vigorously you do an activity (exercise intensity)

cose-lowering effect that results from doing activity, and it can contribute to lack of progress with weight loss efforts.

If you have type 2 diabetes and you take certain types of diabetes pills, you may be at a higher—yet still moderate—risk of experiencing low blood glucose levels with activity. Some, but not all, diabetes pills increase your risk of experiencing hypoglycemia when you exercise (see Table 6-2). If you take one of the medications that puts you at a higher risk, you should be aware of the signs and symptoms of hypoglycemia (see Table 6-3), how to treat it correctly (see Figure 6-1) with carbohydrate (CHO) sources (see Table 6-4), and what actions to take to prevent such lows from happening again.

- *A key point to remember*: If you are trying to lose weight, routinely eating extra food and carbohydrate when exercising can limit your success and can prevent long-term improvements in blood glucose control as you increase activity. However, you should be prepared with carbohydrate foods to treat low blood glucose when you are

TABLE 6-2 Oral Diabetes Medications and Hypoglycemia Risk with Activity

ORAL MEDICATIONS THAT DO INCREASE RISK OF HYPOGLYCEMIA	ORAL MEDICATIONS THAT DON'T INCREASE RISK OF HYPOGLYCEMIA

First-generation sulfonylureas
  Chlorpropamide (Diabinese®)
  Tolazamide (Tolinase®)
  Tolbutamide (Orinase®)
Second-generation sulfonylureas
  Glyburide (DiaBeta®, Micronase®, Glynase Prestabs®)
  Glipizide (Glucotrol®/Glucotrol XL®)
  Glimepiride (Amaryl®)
Meglitinide
  Repaglinide (Prandin®)
	Alpha-glucosidase inhibitors[a,b]
	  Acarbose (Precose®)
	  Miglitol (Glycet®)
	Biguanides[c]
	  Metformin (Glucophage®)
	Thiazolidinediones[a,c]
	  Rosiglitazone (Avandia®)
	  Pioglitazone (Actos®)

[a] Can contribute to hypoglycemia if used as combination therapy with insulin or sulfonylureas.
[b] Glucose must be used as treatment for hypoglycemia; alpha-glucosidase inhibitors prevent sucrose (table sugar) from being an effective treatment.
[c] Hypoglycemia is possible with long duration exercise.

Table 6-3 Signs and Symptoms of Hypoglycemia

- Blood glucose reading of 70 mg/dl or less on your meter*
- Sweating/ changes in body temperature†
- Trembling
- Tingling
- Difficulty concentrating/ thinking slowly
- Lightheadedness/ dizziness
- Slurred speech
- Blurred vision
- Lack of coordination
- Tiredness, fatigue, sleepiness
- Pounding heart/ fast pulse†
- Heavy or rapid breathing†
- Hunger
- General feeling that "something's not right"

*A blood glucose value of 70 mg/dl or less indicates hypoglycemia; always test when you note other symptoms.
† Note these symptoms of hypoglycemia may be "masked" with physical activity because they also result from doing exercise.

active. If you suspect that your blood glucose is too low, test to verify this before eating. It is best to monitor your blood glucose before and after doing activity if you experience unexpected glucose fluctuations. If you find you often have to eat extra foods due to hypoglycemia consider these other options:

- Talk to your physician to make sure the dosages of your medications and the times that you take them are correctly adjusted.
- Consider changing the time of day you exercise in relation to your typical meal and snack times. For example, plan an activity session one or two hours after a meal instead of after a long period of time without food.

If you have type 1 diabetes or type 2 diabetes that is treated with insulin therapy, there is a valid possibility that your blood glucose levels will fall too low with activity. It is very important for you to know the symptoms of hypoglycemia (see Table 6-3), the steps to take to treat lows (see Figure 6-1) with appropriate carbohydrate (CHO) sources

FIGURE 6-1 How to Handle Hypoglycemia with Activity

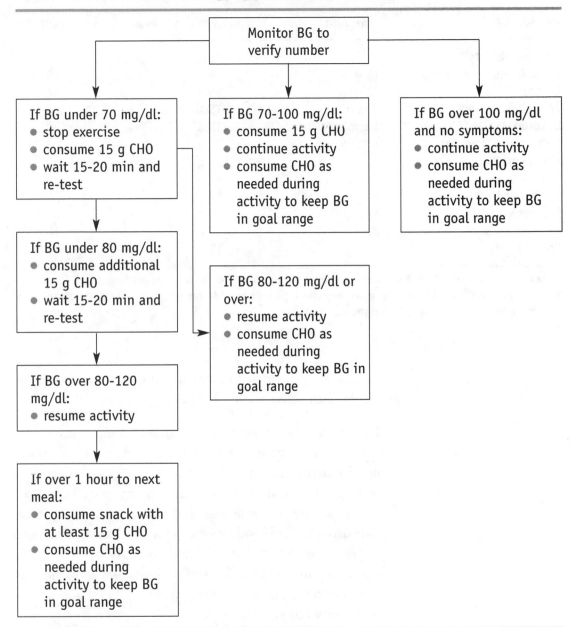

Monitor BG to verify number

If BG under 70 mg/dl:
- stop exercise
- consume 15 g CHO
- wait 15-20 min and re-test

If BG under 80 mg/dl:
- consume additional 15 g CHO
- wait 15-20 min and re-test

If BG over 80-120 mg/dl:
- resume activity

If over 1 hour to next meal:
- consume snack with at least 15 g CHO
- consume CHO as needed during activity to keep BG in goal range

If BG 70-100 mg/dl:
- consume 15 g CHO
- continue activity
- consume CHO as needed during activity to keep BG in goal range

If BG 80-120 mg/dl or over:
- resume activity
- consume CHO as needed during activity to keep BG in goal range

If BG over 100 mg/dl and no symptoms:
- continue activity
- consume CHO as needed during activity to keep BG in goal range

Key: BG = blood glucose; CHO = carbohydrate; g = grams
©2000, The American Dietetic Association. *Sports Nutrition: A Guide for the Professional Working with Active People.* Adapted with permission.

Table 6-4 Carbohydrate (CHO) Sources for Treating Hypoglycemia with Activity

CHO SOURCE	AMOUNT	CHO GRAMS (G.) SUPPLIED	CALORIES*
Glucose Tablets™	3	15 g	60
Insta Glucos™	18 g	15 g	60
Glutose™	40 g	15 g	64
Fruit Juice	½ cup	15 to 20 g	60-80
Gatorade®	1 cup	12 g	50
Soft Drinks (Regular)	½ to ⅔ cup	15 g	55-60
Lifesavers®	8	15 g	60
Gum Drops	6	15 g	65
Fruit Roll-Up®	1	12 g	50
Raisins	2 Tbsp	17 g	75
NutraGrain Bar®	½	15 g	70
Power Bar®	⅓	15 g	60

Note: Be aware that all sources of carbohydrate supply calories. Be aware of portion sizes! Overconsuming (or overtreating hypoglycemia) may cause blood sugars to be elevated later on and can prevent long-term success with weight loss.

(see Table 6-4), and measures to take to prevent hypoglycemia with activity from happening again.

- *A key point to remember*: Blood glucose monitoring before and after activity sessions will help you learn how your blood glucose changes with activity. It will also help you make good decisions about when to exercise based on your blood glucose readings. Remember to test any time you suspect your blood glucose is low so that you can take proper steps to treat hypoglycemia quickly and correctly. If you take insulin or SFU (sulfonylureas), it is possible to develop exercise-induced hypoglycemia several hours after the activity has ended.
- Always be prepared with carbohydrate sources to treat hypoglycemia. If you do vigorous or prolonged activity, lasting more than about 45 minutes, you may need to take in extra carbohydrate every once in a while to keep your blood glucose level in a good range. An intake of 15 to 30 grams of carbohydrate every 15 to 30 minutes of activity is usually enough to keep blood glucose levels

from falling too low. Blood glucose monitoring can help you make good decisions about whether or not you need to eat additional carbohydrate. Remember that overeating can prevent improvements in blood glucose levels and can supply unnecessary calories.

- Know when the insulin you take is peaking, or most actively lowering your blood glucose (Table 6-5). Exercise increases blood flow, which may increase how fast your insulin goes to work. If you exercise when insulin is peaking, you are more likely to experience a large drop in your glucose level than if you exercise before or after peak insulin times.

- If you often experience low blood sugars with activity or you find that you need to consume a lot of extra carbohydrate to keep your blood glucose in a good range, your insulin dosage(s) may need adjusting. Talk to your physician about this.

In summary, when you have diabetes, and particularly when you take diabetes pills or insulin, you must learn how to fit activity into your daily routine for the best possible blood glucose control. For greatest success, activity should be incorporated into a total plan for diabetes management. That means the activity you do and other aspects of diabetes management—including meal planning, medications, stress management and relaxation, and blood glucose monitoring—should complement one another. A skill called pattern management can help you learn how to fit activity into your diabetes care plan.

Table 6-5 Insulin Time/Action Profiles

TYPE OF INSULIN	ONSET	PEAK	DURATION
Insulin lispro	<15 min	1-2 hr	3-4 hr
Regular	0.5-1 hr	2-3 hr	6-8 hr
NPH/Lente	2-4 hr	7-8 hr	10-16 hr
Ultralente	4-6 hr	18 hr	24-36 hr
Insulin glargine	1-2 hr	Has no peak	24 hr

Tailoring Your Diabetes Care Plan

What should your blood glucose levels be? Ideally, they should be in a goal range that you and your diabetes care provider decide is best for you. We know that the risk of developing diabetes complications is reduced when blood glucose levels are kept as close to normal as possible. Desirable target ranges are:

- 80 to 120 mg/dl pre-meal
- 100 to 140 mg/dl at bedtime
- 180 mg/dl or less one hour after a meal
- 150 mg/dl or less two hours after a meal

To keep your blood glucose levels in these ranges once you start to exercise will require some fine-tuning of your diabetes care plan. You may hit on just the right balance immediately, or it may take some time to adjust your plan to fit in with your increased activity. Pattern management is a problem-solving approach that can help you make decisions about how to best control your blood glucose levels. These are the steps of pattern management:

1. **Gather information**
   A. Monitor your blood glucose, and keep a record of your readings.
   B. Make note of variables that may influence your blood glucose levels, including:
      - diabetes medications that you take, their dosages, and when you take them in relation to the time of day that you do activity
      - the timing of activity sessions in relation to when you eat meals and snacks
      - what foods you eat for meals and snacks
      - stress and other factors that may affect blood glucose values on a given day and how they change with activity

2. Study the information that you collect

A. See if you can find repeating patterns or trends in how your blood glucose levels change with activity. A pattern is a series of blood glucose values that, over a period of three to five days, is repeatedly either above, below, or within your goal range at about the same time of day.

B. Look for reasons that explain how blood glucose levels change with activity.

3. Use the information you collect to take action

A. Consider if your diabetes management plan needs adjustment and discuss this with your diabetes care provider; helpful adjustments may include:

- changing the time of day that you do physical activity
- increasing or decreasing how much activity you do
- changing the timing of your meals or snacks in relation to activity
- modifying the amounts or types of foods that you eat before, during, or after doing activity
- changing timing or dosages of medication(s)

B. Try out modified management strategies.

4. Evaluate your action to correct out-of-range blood glucose patterns

A. Continue the steps of pattern management to evaluate how your blood glucose changes with activity once you have modified your management system.

Record keeping is an important part of pattern management. Figure 6-2 is a *Diabetes and Physical Activity Record* that provides an outline for collecting important information that will help you identify blood glucose patterns and achieve blood glucose goals with activity. To illustrate this process, let's look at how Leo, a 52 year old man who has had type 2 diabetes for 3 years, used this record to get a handle on his blood glucose patterns and optimize his diabetes control with activity.

Figure 6-2 Daily Diabetes and Physical Activity Record

Name: _____   Diabetes Medications: _____ (dosage/time)
_____ (dosage/time)

Blood Glucose Goals: *Before meals* _____   *After meals* _____   *Bedtime* _____

DAY	ACTIVITY RECORD			BG RECORD							OTHER/NOTES
-----	------	------	--------	-----------	------	-------	------	-------	------	-------	
				BREAKFAST		LUNCH		DINNER			
	TYPE	TIME	EFFORT	BEFORE	AFTER	BEFORE	AFTER	BEFORE	AFTER		
Mon.											
Tues.											
Wed.											
Thurs.											
Fri.											
Sat.											
Sun.											

FOOD NOTES:

BREAKFAST: Time _____   LUNCH: Time _____   DINNER: Time _____   SNACK: Time _____

Mon.

Tues. _____ _____ _____

Wed. _____ _____ _____

Thurs. _____ _____ _____

Fri. _____ _____ _____

Sat. _____ _____ _____

Sun. _____ _____ _____

KEY INSTRUCTIONS

Diabetes Medications: Note what diabetes medications you take, dosages, and time(s) that you take them.

Blood Glucose Goals: Write down your schedule for blood glucose monitoring and your goals at each time.

Day: Under the day of the week note the date.

Activity Record: Note each session of activity that you do.
  Type: Note the form of activity that you do, for example walking, stretching, or yard work.
  Time: Note the time of day that you do an activity and the duration of each session, for example: 8:30 to 9:00 a.m. walked for 30 min.
  Effort: Use Perceived Exertion (see Chapter 4, Figure 4-1) to identify how hard or difficult the activity seemed while you were doing it.

Blood Glucose Record: Note blood glucose values before and/or two hours after your meal(s). Talk to your doctor or health care team about monitoring and the best schedule for you to follow especially if you are unsure when you should test. Draw a *circle* around any BG that is *below* and a *square* around any BG that is *above* your goal range.

Other: Note any factors or variances, like stress, time of day that you do an activity, illness, or food, that may influence your blood glucose readings. Note results of any additional blood glucose tests that you do, for example, before and after activity.

Food Notes: Note the time(s) of your meals and snacks—especially in relation to exercise times and any variances from your usual way of eating (for example eating more or less than usual, eating later or earlier than usual, or eating foods that are "unusual" for you).

Getting on track— Leo's records

Leo monitored his blood glucose two or three times every day, took his diabetes medications, and attempted to follow a meal plan. However, he did not keep records of his diabetes management. He recently had an appointment with his doctor and found that his HbA1C was higher than he would like at 7.8 percent and that he had gained a few pounds. Leo and his physician discussed benefits of gradually increasing daily physical activity, and Leo decided he would like to work up to doing 30 minutes of activity each day. He wanted to see if this would improve his blood glucose control and help with his efforts to lose some weight. He and his doctor also talked about doing blood glucose monitoring four times per day for a while and keeping a record so that Leo, with the support of diabetes educators, could identify blood glucose patterns and ways to include activity into his diabetes management regime for improved control.

He gathered information

Leo used the *Daily Physical Activity Record* to gather information about his diabetes management. He noted:

- the diabetes medications that he took, including dosages and times
- his blood glucose goals
- the types of activities that he did, the time of day, the amount of time of each activity session, and the perceived effort
- his blood glucose readings from his meter
- factors that may have explained blood glucose readings
- variances in his food intake

He studied the information he collected

Leo then looked at the information he collected. He drew a square around every blood glucose reading that was above his goal range. He found no readings that were below his goal range, but if he had, he would have drawn a circle around these. These are the patterns that Leo identified:

- His blood glucose tended to be elevated in the mornings, both before breakfast and two hours after his meal. When he did morning activity, his morning values improved.

- Two hours after lunch his blood glucose tended to be in his goal range.
- His evening blood glucose—which he, on alternate days, either measured two hours after his meal or at bedtime—was elevated when he did not do evening activity. Stress and overeating may have been contributing factors. He found that staying with his meal plan was most challenging at dinnertime and in the evening.

He used the information to take action

Based on the information that he collected and the blood glucose patterns that he identified, Leo decided to try the following strategies to improve his control:

- get up early and do 15 minutes or more of walking each morning
- do at least 15 minutes of evening activity (either walking, yard work, or another type)
- re-focus on staying with his meal plan in the evening; do some activity or get busy with something else to prevent unnecessary snacking

He evaluated the effectiveness of these new management strategies

Leo continued to keep records, and when he examined them he found that his blood glucose control improved when he increased his amount of activity and better managed his food intake. He found that keeping records increased his self-awareness and was actually very motivational! His follow-up appointment with the diabetes educator was also beneficial because he was able to bring his records, and the very useful information in them, to this visit.

Now, you are aware of guidelines and strategies that can help you achieve and maintain optimal blood glucose control with activity. The guidelines that have been presented are general and the strategies are suggestions of techniques to try. Both are meant to provide you with a foundation and a starting point. However, you have your own history with diabetes and your own physical activity goals. Just how you decide to fit activity into your daily routine is unique to you. Pattern management is a skill that can help you develop and

Figure 6-3 Leo's Record

Daily Diabetes and Physical Activity Record

Name: Leo

Diabetes Medications: *Glipizide (dosage/time) 10 mg 7:30 a.m. 5 mg 6:00 p.m.*
Metformin (dosage/time) 500 mg 3 times/day before meals

Blood Glucose Goals: *Before meals 80 to 120*   *After meals (2 hr) under 150*   *Bedtime 100 to 140*

DAY	ACTIVITY RECORD			BG RECORD						OTHER/NOTES
	TYPE	TIME	EFFORT	BREAKFAST		LUNCH		DINNER		
				BEFORE	AFTER	BEFORE	AFTER	BEFORE	AFTER	
Mon.	walk—car to office	8:30 to 8:40 a.m.	3 moderate	152	175		133		201 (B)	large dinner & dessert
Tues.	walk	8:35 to 8:45 a.m.	3 moderate	126	139		149		188 (2 hr)	stressed! p.m. snack
Wed.	walk	7:05 to 7:20 a.m.	3 moderate	117	143		140		107 (B)	snack at bedtime
	mowed lawn	7:00 to 8:10 p.m.	4 somewhat strong							
Thurs.	walk	6:55 to 7:15 a.m.	3 moderate	119	135		153		211 (2 hr)	dinner out
Fri.	walk	7:00 to 7:30 p.m.	3 moderate	132	181		147		141 (B)	
Sat.	yard work	10:00 to 11:00 a.m.	3 moderate	144	171		92		133 (2 hr)	active day

walk	7:15 to 7:35 p.m.	3		moderate			relaxed	
Sun.	park/play with grandchildren	4:00 to 5:30 p.m.	2-3 weak to moderate	129	135	193	126 (B)	brunch active afternoon

FOOD NOTES:

	BREAKFAST: 8:00 A.M.	LUNCH: 12:30 P.M.	DINNER: 6:30 TO 7:00 P.M.	SNACK:
Mon.	usual	usual	large potato & portion of meat, 1/2 slice cheesecake	none
Tues.	usual	usual	usual	cheese & 12 crackers (5:30 p.m.)
Wed.	usual	usual	usual	popcorn (3 cups) (10:00 p.m.)
Thurs.	usual	usual	large serving pasta & extra slice of bread	none
Fri.	usual	usual	usual	none
Sat.	usual	chips with sandwich	usual	none
Sun.	1 slice toast only	11:00 a.m. brunch combined breakfast/lunch	usual	small cookie (4:30 p.m.)

fine-tune your methods of doing this for long-term success with achieving the best possible diabetes control.

Other Exercise Safety Considerations

Every physical activity session should be a safe and enjoyable experience! That said, there are a few exercise safety considerations that everyone with diabetes should know. These are especially important for anyone who has diabetes complications.

Making good activity choices, especially if you have complications or physical limitations, is a first step toward exercise safety. *Table 1-1: Exercising Safely with Diabetes Complications* identifies activities that are good for you and those you'll have to be cautious about doing when you have complications. Always talk to your doctor if you are not sure if an activity is safe for you to do.

Beyond choosing proper and safe activities, there are additional safety tips that you should follow whenever you are active. Although most of these points require a little attention and pre-planning, they don't require a lot of time and effort. Even so, they contribute significantly to exercise safety. Some of these are sensible for anyone who exercises; others are specific to individuals with diabetes.

General safety points:
- always warm up your muscles at the beginning of an activity session and cool down at the end
- keep exercise intensity (or effort) at a moderate and comfortable level
- avoid doing activity in extremely hot or cold temperatures—choose indoor options when the weather is extreme
- drink at least 2 cups of fluid within two hours of starting exercise and drink fluids often during activity (try to drink ½ to 1 cup of fluid every 15 minutes)
- wear good quality footwear that is appropriate for the activity you plan to do. Shoes with silica gel or air mid-soles are a good choice for weight-bearing activities like walking because they are built to reduce stress on the feet and joints

- wear clothing that is appropriate for the exercise climate (warm in the winter, cool in the summer)
- stop doing an activity if you feel any pain, discomfort, shortness of breath, or light-headedness; report unusual symptoms to your doctor

Diabetes-specific safety points:
- always wear diabetes identification
- always have access to a meter and carry a treatment for hypoglycemia
- monitor blood glucose before and after your exercise routine to evaluate the effects of the activity on your blood glucose levels
- inform someone that you have diabetes and tell them what to do to help you if your blood glucose drops too low during an activity session
- carefully inspect your feet for blisters, redness, or other signs of irritation both before and after doing activity
- wear clean socks (if possible, polyester or cotton/polyester blend) that fit smoothly into your shoe

Become more aware through activity

One of the great things about physical activity is that it is a healthy habit, and it tends to help us focus on other lifestyle habits that contribute to overall health. When we do activity we are clued in to how we feel—great, energetic, sluggish, tired—and this causes us to evaluate why we feel a given way. Many athletes—runners, for example—keep weekly logs of how they feel during workouts and take note of the things that occurred that may have affected their performance. They use this information to fine-tune their training methods and create a competitive edge.

Being physically active when you have diabetes can take some extra effort, especially at first. But like the athlete, keeping a log of your diabetes management and physical activity can be very helpful. Blood glucose monitoring, record keeping, and learning to identify blood glucose patterns are skills that will help you fine-tune strategies for successfully increasing activity in your daily routine. As you go about this process, you will find that you become more and more aware of the foods that you eat, the medications that you take, stress levels, and other factors that influence how you feel and how your blood glucose changes with activity. The benefit of this new awareness is that it can help you to make additional positive lifestyle changes that add to being physically active. You will find yourself, in many ways, being surprisingly persistent about caring for yourself and your diabetes. Through doing physical activity you begin to take charge and successfully self-manage your diabetes for optimal control, improved health, and a heightened sense of well being.

7 Your Fitness Prescription
Some Sample Exercises

Sit, Stretch, and Strengthen

Now that you've seen how easy it is to add a little activity into your daily routine—activity that counts—you might be ready for something a little more structured. The following is an activity routine that can help you gain total body strength and flexibility. The stretching and strengthening activities are designed so that you can do them in your own home, even while you watch TV, enjoy music, or listen to the radio. The routine is broken into three segments, and takes about 30 minutes to complete. But, if you are short on time or are just beginning to do physical activity, you can do just one or two of the segments.

The routine works three separate areas of the body: the upper body, which includes shoulders, chest, and arms; the torso, which takes in the abdominal and back muscles; and the lower body, which includes the hips, legs, ankles, and feet.

If you are new to physical activity, you may want to start off by just doing one or two of these segments, especially if the full routine is more than you are physically able to do at first. For example, on Monday you might do the upper body stretch and strengthen segment; on Tuesday, the torso segment; and on Wednesday, the lower body segment. Then repeat the individual segments on the following days. Another option is to do the *15-Minute Busy Day Routine.* This routine works out those muscles and joints that are typically underused as we go about our daily tasks and are prone to weakness and tightness.

Your Exercise "Equipment"

To get started, all you really need is a strong, stable chair, preferably without arms. Once you can comfortably perform the strengthening exercises, however, you have the option of adding resistance in the form of an elastic band or light weights. These will help challenge your muscles and help you continue to build strength.

When you choose your "equipment," keep these points in mind:

- **A sturdy chair.** The chair should firmly support your back and the seat should be wide enough and deep enough so that you are well supported and can sit comfortably. Your feet should fully rest on the floor and you should be able to position your knees comfortably over the front edge of the seat. The back of the chair should be tall enough that you can stand and hold onto it without bending or hunching over.
- **An exercise band (optional).** The exercise band should be long enough so that you can work against it for resistance but still do the exercises with good posture and form.
- **Weights (optional).** Small hand-held weights, such as dumbbells, will also add resistance to your workout. But canned goods from your pantry can serve the same purpose. Just be sure you can hold the cans comfortably in your hands. To add resistance during leg exercises, purchase weights that strap on to your ankles (see discussion on weights below).

Adding weights to your workout

When you first begin doing strengthening activities, simply lifting your limbs in the air will probably be enough of a workout. As you become stronger, however, you may want to invest in some light weights. This way, you can gradually increase the amount of work you do and continue to strengthen your muscles.

Hand-held weights

Dumbbells are short bars with weights fastened to each end. They typically weigh anywhere from 1 pound to 20 pounds.

To start, invest in just one or two sets of dumbbells. As you gain strength, you might want to buy heavier weights as needed. Another option is to buy a set of adjustable dumbbells. Extra pounds can be added to or subtracted from these weights as you gain strength or to adjust the weight you need to use for a particular exercise. They are fairly inexpensive and don't require much storage space. Dumbbells that are covered with Neoprene are a nice option. The covering makes the weight comfortable to hold and easy to grip.

A cheap and easy alternative to dumbbells is to use canned goods or bottled water in a plastic container as your weights. The latter option is nice because it allows you to add or subtract weight by varying the amount of water in the container. Be certain that you can firmly hold onto any can, bottle, or other container that you use as a weight alternative; it should not be awkward to handle.

Although you may see people carrying hand weights while they are walking or jogging, this is not recommended. Carrying weights can interfere with the way your body should move and can actually cause injury.

Ankle weights

Ankle weights are padded or cushioned cuffs that wrap around your ankles and fasten securely with a strap. The cuff should not cause any rubbing or pressure points and ideally should be constructed of a smooth fabric that breathes.

The weights typically weigh anywhere from 2 to 10 pounds. The most flexible option is to purchase a set of ankle weights with pouches or straps that hold weight bars. Weight bars can then be added or subtracted to increase or decrease weight as needed.

Ankle weights are meant to provide resistance during strengthening exercises. Never use them when you are going out for a walk; they can cause joint injuries.

Increasing the amount of weight you lift

If you have been making progress and gaining strength, you will find that you can lift more weight. Muscles become stronger by lifting heavier loads. When you are able to do 12 to 15 lifts easily and comfortably, you are ready to increase the amount of weight you lift. Start by adding just one pound.

Since you will now be lifting a heavier amount of weight, you will probably need to cut back the number of lifts you do. For example, if you have been doing 12 lifts easily, you may have to cut back to six or eight lifts when you add a 1-pound weight. Gradually work back up to doing 12 to 15 lifts before you add weight again.

Sit, Stretch, and Strengthen Routine

The routine below consists of a warm-up, three exercise segments, and a cool-down. You can do any one segment, two, or all three at an exercise session, but be sure to include the warm-up and cool-down whenever you exercise.

When performing the stretching and strengthening exercises that follow, keep a few tips in mind:

- Do the exercises slowly and with controlled movements. Pay attention to your body position during each exercise.
- Remember to breathe during the exercises. A general rule of thumb when lifting is to exhale on the exertion and inhale on the release. For example, during a side lateral raise you would exhale as you bring your arms out to the side, and inhale as you lower them. During a stretch, focus on breathing deeply and slowly.
- Think about the muscle you are working as you do the stretching or strengthening exercise and perform the exercise in a controlled yet vigorous and active way.

Warm-up   Before you begin the strengthening and stretching routine, do at least a five minute warm-up. A good warm-up increases blood flow to your muscles and joints before you begin any activity. This will allow you to complete the routine comfortably, will reduce your risk of "pulling a muscle," and will maximize the benefit you gain from the strengthening and stretching activities. Here are ideas of ways you can warm up at home:

- march in place while you watch TV
- take a quick walk around your house
- go up and down your stairs at a moderate pace
- turn on some music and dance!

Stretch and Strengthen

Upper body: shoulders, chest, and arms

1. Neck and shoulder stretch

Sit up straight with your back supported by the chair and your arms down at your sides. Gently tilt your head forward toward your chest and hold for 5 seconds. Slowly roll your head to the right, bringing your right ear toward your right shoulder; hold for 5 seconds. Then roll your head forward and to the left, bringing your left ear toward your left shoulder; hold for 5 seconds. Repeat 3 to 5 times.

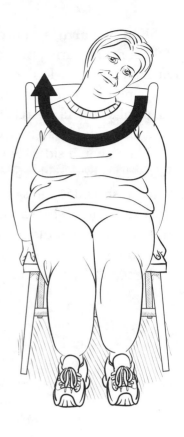

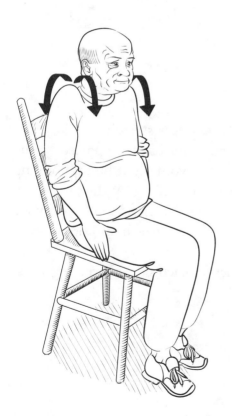

2. Shoulder shrugs

With your arms down at your sides, raise your shoulders toward your ears and slowly roll them forward and down. Repeat 5 to 8 times.

Then raise your shoulders toward your ears and slowly roll them backward and down. Repeat 5 to 8 times.

3. Shoulder, arm, and neck stretch

Hold your right arm just above the elbow with your left hand. As you look over your right shoulder, slowly pull your arm in and toward your left shoulder until you feel a stretch in your shoulder and upper arm. Hold the stretch for 10 seconds.

Then switch sides, holding your left arm just above the elbow with your right hand. Look over your left shoulder and slowly pull your arm in and toward your right shoulder until you feel a stretch in your shoulder and upper arm. Hold for 10 seconds.

Repeat 3 times on each side.

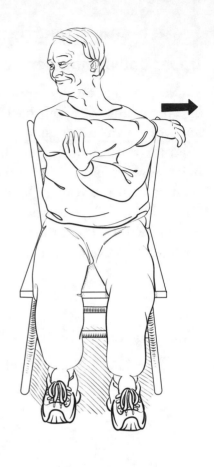

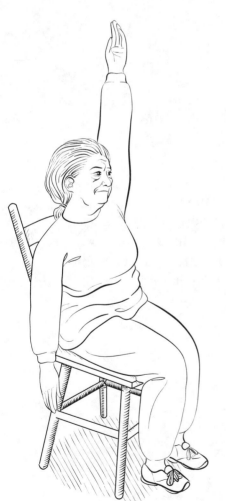

4. Reach high, reach low stretch

Sit up straight with your back supported by the chair. Reach up with your right hand, pointing your fingers toward the ceiling. At the same time, reach down with your left hand and point your fingers toward the floor. Stretch and hold for 10 seconds.

Repeat 5 times for each side, alternating arms.

5. Triceps shoulder stretch

Reach behind your head with your left hand; place it at the top of your back between your shoulder blades. With your right hand, exert slow and gentle pressure on your left elbow until you feel a stretch in the triceps muscle, which runs under your arm from shoulder to elbow. Hold for 10 seconds. Switch sides, placing your right hand at the top of your back and exerting gentle pressure on the right elbow with your left hand.

Repeat 3 times on each side, alternating arms.

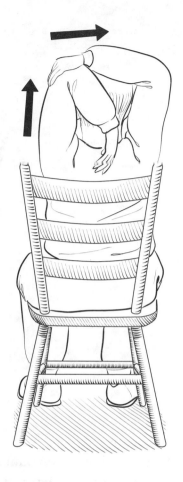

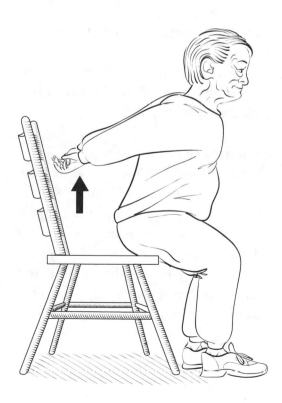

6. Arm, chest, shoulder stretch

Sit forward in your chair with your back straight and feet firmly on the floor. Clasp your hands behind your back, just above your seat. Take a deep breath in and, keeping your elbows slightly bent, slowly "pull" your arms upward until you feel a stretch across the chest and in the arms and shoulders. Breathe naturally and think about lifting your chest upward as you stretch. Hold the stretch for 10 seconds.

Repeat 3 times.

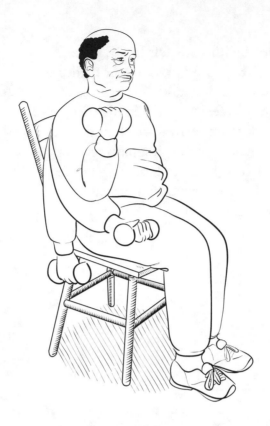

7. Biceps curl

Sit up straight with your back supported by the chair. Grasp a weight in each hand and lower your arms to your sides with your palms facing in. With your upper arms and elbows held in close to your sides, bend your elbow to curl the weight in your left hand up to thigh level. Now rotate your hand to a palm-up position and continue to slowly bend your elbow until the weight reaches shoulder level.

Now slowly lower the weight, palm up, to thigh level. Rotate your palm so that it faces your thigh, straighten your elbow, and return the weight to the starting position.

Repeat the lift 8 to 12 times (or as many repetitions as you find comfortable), then switch arms.

Key points to remember.

- For all lifting activities use slow, controlled movements (count slowly 1,2,3,4,5 as you lift, and then repeat the count as you bring the weight down).
- Exhale as you lift the weight and inhale as you return your arm to the starting position.

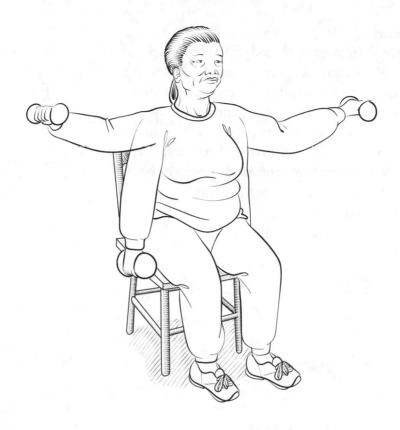

8. Side lateral raise

Sit forward in your chair with your feet firmly on the floor. Grasp a weight in each hand and lower your arms to your sides with your palms facing in. Keeping your elbows slightly bent, slowly raise both arms out to the side until your hands are just above shoulder level. (This is your goal; if you cannot reach to shoulder level, simply lift to a comfortable position for you.) Pause, then slowly lower your arms to the starting position. Remember to exhale as you lift the weight and inhale as you lower it.

Repeat 8 to 12 times.

- If raising both arms at the same time is too difficult, try this method: Keeping your body straight in the chair, hold onto the side of your chair with one hand. With a weight in the other hand, do 8 to 12 lifts, then switch and do the exercise with the opposite arm.

9. Triceps curl

Sit up straight with your back supported by the chair; look straight ahead and keep your chin parallel to the floor. Holding a weight in your left hand, raise it above your head; keep your arm straight, with the elbow facing forward and your upper arm close to your head. With your right hand, grasp the back of your left upper arm for support, just above the elbow. Slowly bend your elbow and lower the weight toward your left shoulder. Return to the starting position.

Do 8 to 12 repetitions with your left arm then switch arms.

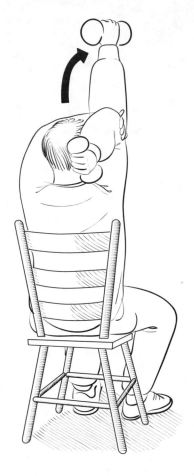

10. Seated chest fly (performed with exercise band)

Sit up straight with your back supported by the chair. Hold one end of an exercise band in each hand and raise your arms straight up over your head. Now lower the band behind your head and position it across your back, just below your shoulder blades. Keeping your elbows slightly bent, straighten your arms out to either side and slowly bring your arms forward until your forearms meet in front of your chest. Exhale as you bring the arms in, and inhale as you slowly return your arms out to the side.

Repeat 8 to 12 times.

Torso: abdominals and back

11. Side stretch

Sit up straight in your chair, with the hips slightly forward from the chair back and feet placed firmly on the floor. Keeping your hips in a forward position, turn your upper body to the right. As you look over your right shoulder, grasp the chair back and gently pull against it until you feel a stretch in your left side. Hold the stretch for 10 to 15 seconds.

Repeat the stretch 2 to 3 times, alternating sides.

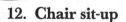

12. Chair sit-up

Sit up straight in your chair with your feet firmly on the floor, arms bent at your sides, and hands in front of your chest with palms facing forward (as if you are going to push something). Slowly bend forward at the waist, pulling in your abdominal muscles and keeping your back straight. As you bend forward, extend your elbows and push out with your hands, exhaling as you go. Slowly come up and return to the starting position.

Repeat 8 to 12 times.

13. Seated abdominal curl

Sit forward in your chair with your hips toward the front edge of the seat. Lean back so that your upper back is supported by the back of the chair. Hold onto the sides of the seat for support and extend your legs out in front of you. Keep your knees slightly bent, heels on the floor, and toes up. Cross your left ankle over your right, pull in your abdominal muscles, and slowly lift your feet 2 to 3 inches off the floor (the effort to lift should come from your abdominal muscles not your hips). Pause, then slowly lower your legs to the starting position.

Repeat for 8 to 12 lifts, then cross your right ankle over your left and repeat.

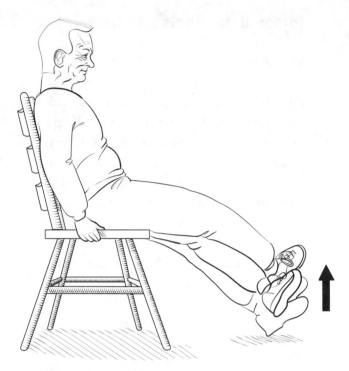

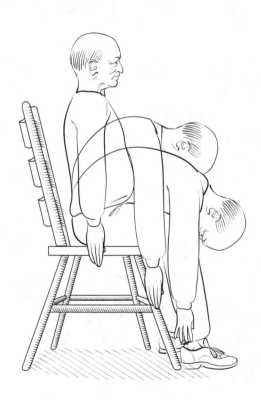

14. Seated lower back/cat stretch

Sit up straight in your chair, feet firmly on the floor. Slowly bend forward, lowering the chest toward your thighs; let your arms dangle toward your feet. Hold the stretch for 10 to 15 seconds, then round your upper back, tuck your chin toward your chest, and lift your upper body half-way to the starting position; continue to let your arms dangle toward your feet. Hold this position for 10 to 15 seconds, then put your hands on your thighs and slowly lift your upper body to the starting position.

Repeat 3 times.

- If you have retinopathy or have been advised to limit head-low activities and posture changes for any other health reason, check with your physician before you do this stretch.

15. Reverse chair sit-up

Sit up straight in your chair, hips at the back of the seat, feet firmly on the floor, and hands lightly gripping the sides of the chair for support. Keeping the back straight, bend forward, chest toward thighs. Slowly straighten up to a seated position with your back supported by the chair.

Repeat 8 to 12 times.

■ To increase the resistance, loop an exercise band under the arches of your feet (always wear shoes!), and hold one end of the band in each hand. Bend your elbows and anchor your hands against your chest, palms in. Now bend forward and then slowly straighten to a seated position with your back supported by the chair. Repeat 8 to 12 times.

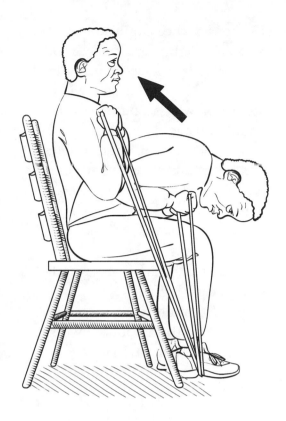

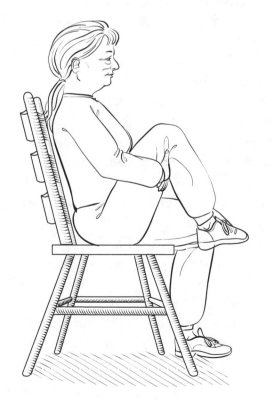

Lower body: hips, legs, ankles, and feet

16. Knee to chest stretch

Sit up straight with your back supported by the chair, feet on the floor. Clasp your hands around your left knee and slowly pull your knee up toward your chest; hold for 10 to 15 seconds.

Repeat 3 times, then switch sides, pulling your right knee toward your chest.

17. Seated knee extension

Sit up straight with your back supported by the chair, feet and knees positioned shoulder-width apart. Slowly straighten your right knee and lift your foot until it is straight out in front of you; flex your ankle and point your toes toward the ceiling. Relax your ankle and slowly lower your leg to the starting position. Repeat with your left leg.

Do 8 to 12 extensions on each side, alternating legs.

- Use ankle weights to increase the amount of work as you gain strength.

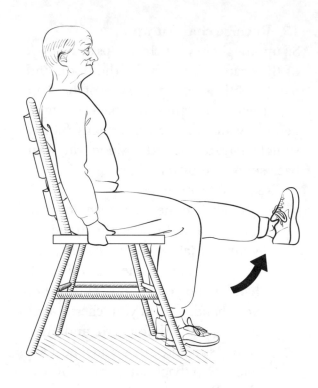

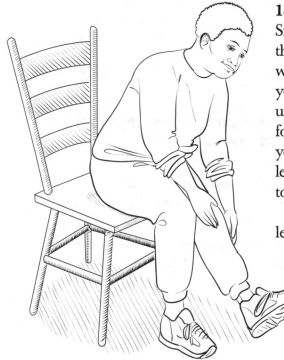

18. Seated hamstring stretch

Sit up straight with your back supported by the chair. Keep your right foot on the floor while you extend your left leg out in front of you with the heel on the floor, toes pointing up. Keeping your back straight, slowly bend forward bringing your upper body toward your left knee. Gently hold your lower left leg with your hands. Hold the stretch for 10 to 15 seconds.

Repeat the stretch 3 times on the left leg, then switch legs.

- If you have been advised to avoid posture changes or "head-low" activities, you may use a foot stool, ottoman, or another chair when you do this stretch. Extend your leg and place the lower leg and heel on the stool or ottoman, toes pointed up. Be certain your leg is well supported.

19. Standing hip extension

Stand about 1½ feet behind your chair and hold onto the back for support. Bend forward at the waist with a slight angle. Look straight ahead, keeping your head, neck, and torso in a straight line. Bend your right knee slightly for support, then slowly lift your left leg behind you until your leg and torso are aligned; your toes should be 8 to 12 inches from the floor and pointed down toward it. Slowly return your leg to the starting position. Repeat, raising your right leg.

Do 8 to 12 lifts on each side, alternating legs.

- You may add ankle weights to increase the amount of work as you gain strength.

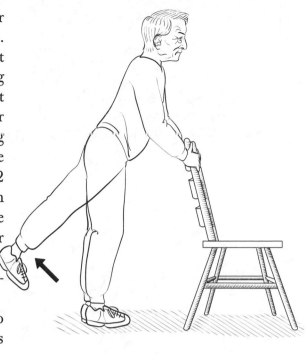

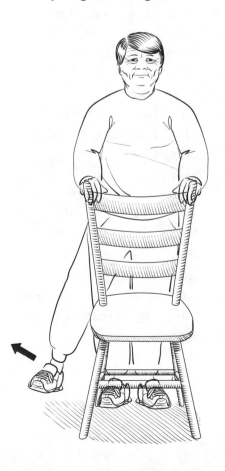

20. Standing side hip raise

Stand 4 to 6 inches behind your chair and hold on to the back for support. Keeping your toes pointed forward and your leg straight, slowly lift your right leg out to the side until it is about 6 inches off the floor. Keep the knee of the supporting leg slightly bent and your torso upright. Pause at the top of the lift, then return your right leg to its starting position.

Do 8 to 12 lifts on each side, alternating legs.

- You may use ankle weights to increase the amount of work as you gain strength.

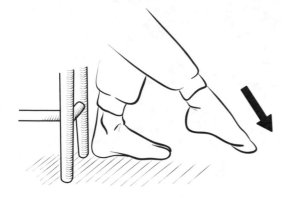

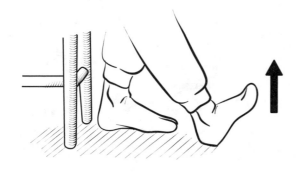

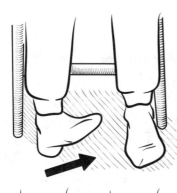

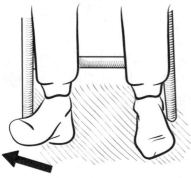

21. Seated foot and toe stretches

A. Sit up straight with your back supported by the chair and your feet on the floor. Lift one heel off the floor, point your toes, and extend them forward and downward until you feel a mild stretch; hold for 10 to 15 seconds. Return to starting position and repeat with the other foot.

B. Rest one heel on the floor, then slowly flex your ankle and pull your toes up so they point toward the ceiling; hold for 10 to 15 seconds. Return to starting position and repeat with the other foot.

C. With your feet flat on the floor, lift the toes of one foot 1 to 2 inches off the floor. Rotate your toes in so they point toward your opposite foot; hold for 10 to 15 seconds. Return to starting position and repeat with the other foot.

D. With your feet flat on the floor, lift the toes of one foot 1 to 2 inches off the floor. Rotate your toes out and away from your other foot; hold for 10 to 15 seconds. Return to starting position and repeat with the other foot.

22. Toe stand

Stand 12 inches behind the back of your chair with your feet shoulder width apart; hold onto the back of the chair for support. Slowly raise your heels off the floor and lift up onto the balls of your feet. Pause, then slowly lower your heels to starting position.

Repeat 8 to 12 times.

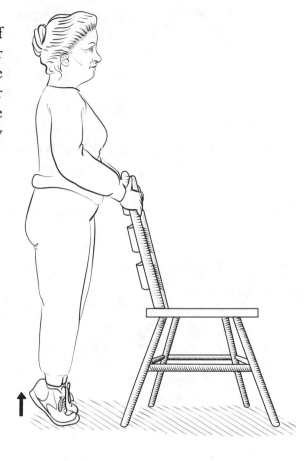

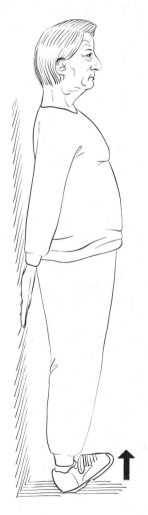

23. Heel stand

For this last exercise, use a wall for support. Stand with your back against the wall, arms down at your sides, and the palms of your hands against the wall. Place your heels a few inches out from the wall, then slowly raise your toes off the floor and balance on your heels. Pause, then slowly lower your toes to the starting position.

Repeat 8 to 12 times.

Cool-down   Just as you began this routine with a warm-up, it is important to end it with a good 5 minute cool-down. The purpose of a cool-down period is to allow your body to gradually get used to a resting state after activity. To cool down, simply repeat a few of the stretches from the sit and stretch routine. This will help minimize any muscle soreness or tightness after you are done. At the end of the cool-down, it is nice to sit back in your chair, close your eyes, take some deep breaths in and out, and focus on how good you feel!

Table 7-1 Sit, Stretch, and Strengthen Summary Sheet

Warm-up (5 minutes)

Stretch and Strengthen

Upper body: shoulders, chest, and arms
1. Neck and shoulder stretch
2. Shoulder shrugs
3. Shoulder, arm, and neck stretch
4. Reach high, reach low stretch
5. Triceps shoulder stretch
6. Arm, chest, shoulder stretch
7. Biceps curl
8. Side lateral raise
9. Triceps curl
10. Seated chest fly

Torso: abdominals and back
11. Side stretch
12. Chair sit-up
13. Seated abdominal curl
14. Seated lower back/cat stretch
15. Reverse chair sit-up

Lower body: hips, legs, ankles, and feet
16. Knee to chest stretch
17. Seated knee extension
18. Seated hamstring stretch
19. Standing hip extension
20. Standing side hip raise
21. Seated foot and toe stretches
22. Toe stand
23. Heel stand

Cool-down (5 minutes)

Tips to remember:

When you stretch:
- Hold the stretch for 10 to 15 seconds
- Focus on relaxed breathing, avoid breath holding
- Keep it comfortable
- Avoid *bouncing* or *bobbing*

When you strengthen:
- Do slow, controlled movements (count 1,2,3,4,5 up/out then 1,2,3,4,5 down/in)
- Focus on breathing (breathe out as you push or lift; breathe in as you return to the relaxed, starting position)
- Keep it comfortable
- Start slowly and gradually build up (The suggested number of repetitions of an exercise are optimal *goals*. If you are not able to do this many at first, start with fewer (4 to 6) repetitions and gradually increase the number that you do. When you feel *mild* muscle discomfort, this is a good indication that you have done enough.)
- Always ask your physician if you are uncertain whether a stretch or strengthening activity is a safe activity for you

Table 7-2 15 Minute Busy Day Routine

Warm-up (5 minutes)

Stretch and Strengthen

Upper body: shoulders, chest, and arms
1. Neck and shoulder stretch
2. Shoulder shrugs
3. Shoulder, arm, and neck stretch
5. Triceps shoulder stretch
8. Side lateral raise
9. Triceps curl

Torso: abdominals and back
11. Side stretch
12. Chair sit-up
14. Seated lower back/cat stretch
15. Reverse chair sit-up

Lower body: hips, legs, ankles, and feet
16. Knee to chest stretch
18. Seated hamstring stretch
19. Standing hip extension
20. Standing side hip raise
21. Seated foot and toe stretches

Cool-down (5 minutes)

APPENDIX

Physical Activity, Diabetes and Health Resources

Organizations, Associations, and Agencies

American Diabetes Association
1701 Beauregard St.
Alexandria, VA 22311
1-800-DIABETES
www.diabetes.org

American Dietetic Association
216 West Jackson Blvd.
Chicago, IL 60606-6995
1-312-899-0040
www.eatright.org

American Heart Association National Center
7272 Greenville Ave.
Dallas, TX 75231-4596
1-888-AHA-USA-1
1-888-MY-HEART
www.amhrt.org

Centers for Disease Control and Prevention
Division of Nutrition and Physical Activity
4770 Buford Hwy. NE (MS-k46)
Atlanta, GA 30341
1-888-232-4674
www.cdc.gov/nccdphp/dnpa

Diabetes Exercise and Sports Association
(formerly International Diabetic Athletes Association)
1647-B West Bethany Home Rd.
Phoenix, AZ 85015-2507
Phone: (602) 433-2113 or 1-800-898-IDAA
Fax: (602) 433-9331
www.diabetes-exercise.org

National Diabetes Information Clearinghouse
1 Information Way
Bethesda, MD 20892-3560
(301) 654-3327
www.niddk.nih.gov

Shape Up America
5707 Democracy Blvd. Suite 305
Bethesda, MD 20817
Fax: (301) 493-9504
www.shapeup.org

Books

ACSM Fitness Book
American College of Sports Medicine
Leisure Press (1992)
A Division of Human Kinetics Publishers
Box 5076
Champaign, IL 61825-5076

American Heart Association Fitting in Fitness:
Hundreds of Simple Ways to Put More Physical Activity into Your Life
American Heart Association (1997)

The American Heart Association Walking Book:
The American Heart Association Walking Program
American Heart Association (1995)

Getting in Shape: Workout Programs for Men and Women
Bob Anderson, Ed Burke, Bill Pearl
Shelter Publications Inc. (1994)
P.O. Box 279
Bolinas, CA 94924
1-800-307-0131

**Living with Exercise: Improving Your Health
Through Moderate Physical Activity**
Steven N. Blair PED
American Health Publishing Company (1991)
The Learn® Education Center
155 W. Mockingbird Ln. Suite 203
Dallas, TX 75235
1-800-736-7323

Strong Women Stay Slim
Miriam E. Nelson PhD
Bantam Doubleday Dell (1999)

Strong Women Stay Young
Miriam E. Nelson, PhD, and Sarah Wernick, PhD
Bantam Doubleday Dell (1998)

Booklets, Brochures and Other Educational Materials

Fitting Fitness In Even When You're Pressed for Time
Education Department
National Cattleman's Beef Association
444 North Michigan Avenue, Suite 1800
Chicago, IL 60611
1-800-368-3138
(specify free offer "ESUA4" when you order)

Eating Smart Even When You're Pressed for Time
Education Department
National Cattleman's Beef Association
444 North Michigan Avenue, Suite 1800
Chicago, IL 60611
1-800-368-3138
(specify free offer "ESUA4" when you order)

On Your Way to Fitness
"On Your Way to Fitness"
P.O. Box 9738
Bridgeport, CT 06699
Send $1.00 with order

99 Tips for Family Fitness Fun
"99 Tips"
c/o MET-Rx Foundation for Health Enhancement
2112 Business Center Dr.
Irvine, CA 92715-1014

Video/Audio Tapes

Beginning fitness / moderate maintenance level:

Armchair Fitness: An Aerobic Workout for People of All Ages
CC-M Productions
7755 16th St. NW
Washington, DC 20012
1-800-453-6280 or (202) 453-6280

Fitness Forever: The Exercise Program for Healthy Aging
(Informative and balanced fitness routine based on sound exercise principles.
 Follows the American College of Sports Medicine Position Stand
Recommendations "Exercise and Physical Activity for Older Adults.")
13820 Donner Pass Rd.
Truckee, CA 96161
1-800-985-5185 or (530) 550-9866
health@telis.org

Gentle Fitness
(Simple activities. Focuses on stretching, easy movement, and relaxation.)
Gentle Fitness Inc.
732 Lake Shore Dr.
Rhinelander, WI 54501
1-800-566-7780 or (715) 362-9260
www.gentlefitness.com

The Healthy Heart Walking Tape: Walking Workouts for a Lifetime of Fitness
Rita Mireno/American Heart Association
Simon & Schuster (Audio) (1996)

Stay in shape/moderate-brisk maintenance level:
These tapes are good options if you have a good "fitness foundation" and are able to walk briskly for about 30 minutes.

Walk Aerobics 40 Plus Workout or 2 Mile Walk with Leslie Sansone
(includes movements that require good balance and agility)
Parade Video/PPI Entertainment Group
Peter Pan Industries Inc.
88 St. Francis St.
Newark, NJ 07105

Web Sites

Questions to ask when evaluating health and fitness information on the internet

- What type of Web site is it?
  - ➢ .com or commercial site (often selling a product or service)
  - ➢ .edu or educational (university or college) site
  - ➢ .gov or government agency site
  - ➢ .org or organization (nonprofit, not for profit or for profit) site

- Who are the authors?
  - ➢ Are they listed?
  - ➢ What are their credentials, including professional certifications and/or licenses?
  - ➢ What is their occupation or employment experience?
  - ➢ Will they gain financially from the information included on the Web site?

Note: authors of .com sites are often trying to sell something and may be financially motivated

- What is the purpose of the web site?
    - ➢ To inform or explain?
    - ➢ To present an opinion or promote a cause?
    - ➢ To persuade?
    - ➢ To sell?

- How reliable is the information included on the site?
    - ➢ Is an original source or reference for the information given?
    - ➢ What is the original source of the information-book, professional journal, magazine, or newspaper?
    - ➢ What institution supports or represents the information-academic institution, government agency, health organization, or private company? Or is this a personal Web page?
    - ➢ How current is the information and when was the site last updated?

Some web sites to investigate:

www.discoverfitness.com
www.fitness.com
www.fitness.org
www.fitnessfind.com
www.fitnesslink.com
www.fitnessworld.com
www.mayohealth.org
www.netsweat.com
www.nih.gov/health/exercise
www.physicalfitness.org
www.primusweb.com/fitnesspartner
www.walkingmag.com
www.webmd.com

(Also note internet addresses for organizations, associations, agencies, and other resources listed in other sections of this appendix.)

Index

C

Carbohydrate (CHO) sources, for treating hypoglycemia with activity, 77

Cardiorespiratory endurance
as a component of fitness, 60
improving, 61

Caring, about exercise, 1–11

Change, deciding in favor of, 19–21

CHO. *See* Carbohydrate sources

Complications, associated with diabetes related diseases, 8

Contracts, making with yourself, 16–18

Cool-down phase, of an exercise session, 68, 108

Costs/benefits of physical activity, balancing, 22

Cues, giving yourself, 21–23

D

Daily Diabetes and Physical Activity Record form, 82–83
sample, 86–87

Daily routine. *See also* Sit, stretch and strengthen routine
establishing, 13–19
extending, 35–36

Diabetes care plan, 80–88
evaluation, 81, 85, 88–89
information gathering, 80–81, 84
record keeping, 80–84
studying information gathered, 81, 84–85
taking action, 81, 85

Diabetes educators, 84

Diabetes medications. *See also* Insulin
effect on hypoglycemia risk with activity, 75

Diabetic ketoacidosis (DKA), 73

Diabetics. *See* People with diabetes

Diet. *See* Eating well

Disease conditions
complications for diabetics with, 8
reasons for consulting physician before beginning exercise, 59

Distorted thoughts, positive alternatives, 20

DKA. *See* Diabetic ketoacidosis (DKA)

Dumbbells, 92–94, 98–100

Duration of exercise, 60–67

E

Eating well, 10

Endurance
cardiorespiratory, 60
muscular, 60

"Equipment" for exercise, 92–93
exercise band, 92, 100, 103
sturdy chair, 92
weights, 92–94, 98–100

Errands. *See also* On the town
exercises you can do, 51–53

Exercise, 31–33, 91–109. *See also* Structured exercises
aerobic, 64
benefits of, 1–7, 22
caring about, 1–11
"equipment" for, 92–94
FITT Principle for, 60–66
reasons for consulting physician before beginning, 59
safety in, 6–8, 29–30, 59, 71–90

Exercise band, 92, 100, 103

Exercise sessions, 67–68
aerobic phase, 67–68
cool-down phase, 68
warm-up phase, 67

About the American Diabetes Association

The American Diabetes Association is the nation's leading voluntary health organization supporting diabetes research, information, and advocacy. Its mission is to prevent and cure diabetes and to improve the lives of all people affected by diabetes. The American Diabetes Association is the leading publisher of comprehensive diabetes information. Its huge library of practical and authoritative books for people with diabetes covers every aspect of self-care—cooking and nutrition, fitness, weight control, medications, complications, emotional issues, and general self-care.

To order American Diabetes Association books: Call 1-800-232-6733. http://store.diabetes.org [Note: there is no need to use **www** when typing this particular Web address]

To join the American Diabetes Association: Call 1-800-806-7801. www.diabetes.org/membership

For more information about diabetes or ADA programs and services: Call 1-800-342-2383. E-mail: Customerservice@diabetes.org www.diabetes.org

To locate an ADA/NCQA Recognized Provider of quality diabetes care in your area: Call 1-703-549-1500 ext. 2202. www.diabetes.org/recognition/Physicians/ListAll.asp

To find an ADA Recognized Education Program in your area: Call 1-888-232-0822. www.diabetes.org/recognition/education.asp

To join the fight to increase funding for diabetes research, end discrimination, and improve insurance coverage: Call 1-800-342-2383. www.diabetes.org/advocacy

To find out how you can get involved with the programs in your community: Call 1-800-342-2383. See below for program Web addresses.

- *American Diabetes Month:* Educational activities aimed at those diagnosed with diabetes-month of November. www.diabetes.org/ADM

- *American Diabetes Alert:* Annual public awareness campaign to find the undiagnosed-held the fourth Tuesday in March. www.diabetes.org/alert

- *The Diabetes Assistance & Resources Program (DAR):* diabetes awareness program targeted to the Latino community. www.diabetes.org/DAR

- *African American Program:* diabetes awareness program targeted to the African American community. www.diabetes.org/africanamerican

- *Awakening the Spirit: Pathways to Diabetes Prevention & Control:* diabetes awareness program targeted to the Native American community. www.diabetes.org/awakening

To find out about an important research project regarding type 2 diabetes: www.diabetes.org/ada/research.asp

To obtain information on making a planned gift or charitable bequest: Call 1-888-700-7029. www.diabetes.org/ada/plan.asp

To make a donation or memorial contribution: Call 1-800-342-2383. www.diabetes.org/ada/cont.asp